KT-567-973

Bernadette Bohan's
The Choice
The Programme

Also by Bernadette Bohan

The Choice

Bernadette Bohan's
The Choice
The Programme

*The simple health plan that saved Bernadette's life –
and could help save yours too*

Bernadette Bohan

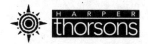

thorsons

HarperThorsons
An Imprint of HarperCollins*Publishers*
77–85 Fulham Palace Road
Hammersmith, London W6 8JB

The website address is: www.thorsonselement.com

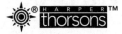

and *HarperThorsons* are trademarks of
HarperCollins*Publishers* Limited

Published by HarperThorsons 2006

7

© Bernadette Bohan 2006

Bernadette Bohan asserts the moral right to
be identified as the author of this work

A catalogue record for this book
is available from the British Library

ISBN-13 978-0-00-722551-4
ISBN-10 0-00-722551-2

Printed and bound in Great Britain by
Clays Ltd, St Ives plc

All rights reserved. No part of this publication may be
reproduced, stored in a retrieval system, or transmitted,
in any form or by any means, electronic, mechanical,
photocopying, recording or otherwise, without the
prior written permission of the publishers.

Mixed Sources
Product group from well-managed
forests and other controlled sources
www.fsc.org Cert no. SW-COC-1806
© 1996 Forest Stewardship Council
FSC

To Ger, Richard, Sarah and Julie
for their love and encouragement

Contents

The Recipes   **119**

Resources   **245**

Bibliography and Recommended Reading   **255**

Index of Recipes   **257**

Acknowledgements

My warmest gratitude to the readers of *The Choice* for their overwhelming feedback on the book and their confirmation that The Programme was helpful for so many.

My heartfelt thanks to my dear friends Deidre, Veronica and Darragh for their friendship and loyalty.

My sincere thanks to Moira Reilly of HarperCollins for her consistent hard work and enthusiasm.

My deep appreciation for my editors Wanda Whiteley and Susanna Abbott of HarperCollins for their support and expertise.

A big thank you to Alex, Karen, Eileen, Gosia, Stephen, David and the chefs at Cornucopia for their valuable input on this project.

A Personal
Introduction

I hope to show you that with some practical basic information you too can live a healthy life without having to become an expert or nutritionist.

The Means to Better Health

This is not rocket science ... keep it simple and just do it!

Rather than concentrating on what you *can't eat*, this book concentrates on what you *can eat*. I feel there is no need to waste time preaching about what you cannot eat, as I strongly believe that nowadays we are bombarded with too much of this kind of negative information. Instead, I find it more useful to suggest that you should add more nourishing foods to your daily routine eating patterns. Furthermore, this way offers you the means to discover that when your body is *nourished*, the constant cravings for junk food and treats will all but disappear. Even if you believe you presently lead a fairly healthy lifestyle, I assure you that nourishing your body further will bring about even more energy, will keep you feeling fantastic, and will culminate in giving you much greater health.

Maybe you are happy with your quality of life, but I suspect the fact that you bought this book means you may not be and you are looking for some sort of change. You may well want to 'clean up your act', but whether your interest in food stems from problems with your health or with maintaining your health, I hope this book will spark your imagination and illustrate how easy these goals are to achieve. I hope to show you how I, an ordinary woman and mother of three, having twice faced cancer, managed to transform my diet and lifestyle without any great hardship. I also hope to show you that with some basic practical information *you too* can live a healthy life without becoming an expert or a nutritionist.

My motivation for writing this book is a direct response to the many requests I received for more information on what I have done to improve my own health. It is also in response to the countless requests for simple and easy-to-follow recipes – recipes for food that can both protect us from disease and comfort and nourish the body. I have included in this book my recommendations surrounding the four changes that I made to my own lifestyle, namely:

- ❖ Juicing fruit and vegetables on a daily basis
- ❖ Introducing powerful foods to my diet daily
- ❖ Cleaning the water coming into my home
- ❖ Switching to safe personal care products.

These changes are simple and easy to implement if you have the motivation to do so. The benefits for me were many and helped me to recover from chemotherapy and radiation cancer treatments. For me the motivation was easy to understand: when diagnosed with cancer for a second time I wanted to find how to treat the cause of the disease and not just the symptoms. I discovered that nutrition plays a big part in combating the effects of degenerative diseases that affect so many of us. Never underestimate the value of good food – it can do more than sustain life! All research, to the highest level of biochemistry, exemplifies the benefits of maintaining health rather than waiting until we have a problem that needs to be fixed.

Nowadays many of us eat for comfort, and believe me I'm all for a bit of comfort, especially living in a cold damp climate like Ireland! There is nothing nicer than a warm soup or a hot dinner on a cold wet windy day, but our bodies have certain requirements that demand we also eat for *nourishment*. When we meet these requirements we get the body's defence mechanisms functioning properly and achieve optimal health.

We can readily accept that machines need oil, fuel and water to run smoothly and to prevent them from breaking down. Likewise it is imperative that we supply the correct fuel to our bodies.

I was touched and impressed with an e-mail I recently received from a 13-year-old girl who, having read my first book *The Choice*, decided that she was going to try to look after her health a little better. This young girl is not much older than my own daughter Julie. She is not suffering from any ill-health and yet has the foresight, common sense and responsibility to want to take care of her health at this young age.

For me, healthy eating has become a great pleasure and has opened up many new tastes and ideas. These simple practical changes are easy to implement in day-to-day life no matter how busy you are, to help you improve your health. Ask yourself:

❖ How often have you stood in the supermarket and wondered what you could buy for yourself and your family that was healthy and did not take hours to prepare?

❖ Have you ever visited a healthfoods store and wanted to buy some wholefoods but you were not quite sure how to prepare them?

Believe me, I know exactly where you're coming from. I now find that having opened up my diet to a much greater variety of foods, many of the foods I used to like now taste rather bland.

My experience has shown me that many of us have become collectors of information. Yet very often we are not prepared to put this information into practice. Remember that actions speak louder than words, and if diagnosed with a life-threatening disease, as I was on two occasions, you no longer have the luxury of time and you soon learn to focus on the job in hand. If only we could use our natural instincts and a little common sense to eat the foods that make us feel good, many of our health problems would disappear.

This is not rocket science – so my method is to keep it simple and JUST DO IT.

You too can also *do it!*

My Story

I was so determined in my quest to beat cancer that I immediately set about making some changes. Whatever the outcome was to be, I was not about to sit around and wait until I got to the point of no return. I had to find a way to help myself.

A Food-fight for Life

When diagnosed with cancer I thought 'Why Me?'
… Well, why not me?

I thought that I had been leading a fairly healthy life. I ate fruit and vegetables every day and I did not overindulge in treats or junk. OK, I'll admit I had a glass of red wine in the evening, but wasn't that meant to be good for me? And yet here I was – facing cancer for a second time round. How could this be happening to me?

My story is in no way unique, nor is it a story of doom and gloom. On the contrary, it is simply the story of an ordinary mother who tried to take responsibility and reshape the life that she so desperately wanted to hold on to. Rather than resigning myself to my fate, I luckily came to realize that where there's a will there's a way.

Eighteen years ago, when I was 33 years of age and married with two small children, I developed cancer of the lymph system. I was pregnant at the time and subsequently lost my baby. I was advised by doctors not to have any more children, as it might well have been the pregnancy hormones that triggered the cancer. At that stage I took the medical advice and treatment and did as I was told. I went home with armfuls of drugs and felt completely helpless.

After seven years free of cancer I believed that I was cured … I made the choice to have another baby. It dawned on me that in the eyes of the medical profession I may have appeared irresponsible, but for me it was a compulsion stronger than sense. I knew I was rocking the boat and that it could well work out to be a reckless decision, possibly jeopardizing my comfortable existence with my two children and husband Ger. The longing for another baby, however, was so deep and instinctive that I decided to take that chance. After all, life is for living, and where would we be in life if we never took any risks?

Unlike my other pregnancies there was no rush of congratulations – it was like I had been selfish and reckless in my decision. My oncologist had been telling me for many years to put the thought of another child out of my mind and that I was better off than most other people as I already had a boy and a girl. Thankfully for us this was one piece of advice I didn't listen to, and the decision turned out to be a blessing. My third child Julie, the joy of all our lives, was born safe and sound. The happy times and everyday dramas of motherhood took over, and concerns about cancer receded into the background of my family life. But, like the predator it is, the cancer was merely biding its time.

Here was I, 12 years after the first time, and the cancer had now returned in my breast. I can still remember back to that first time when my son Richard was seven and my daughter Sarah was only four years old. How frightening it was then, as a young mother looking at my beautiful children, to face the possibility that I might not live to see them grow up! With the same disbelief I experienced on that occasion, I could not believe that I was back in this situation again. Julie was now five, and it was like history repeating itself – *déjà vu!* What had I done to deserve this disease a second time? This was too cruel for one person in one lifetime! If only I'd had the foresight in the first place to learn how to prevent it!

It was then that I decided to get to the bottom of the problem and educate myself. I had to find a way to fight back. By examining the fundamental role of nutrition and diet, I discovered they had a huge role to play in combating the effects of this cruel and frightening disease – a disease which is now affecting one in three women and one in two men in the world today. A number of questions stood at the forefront of my mind:

* Why have so many of us become so susceptible to this deadly disease?
* What made my immune system so weak that it had lost the ability to protect itself?
* Why has conventional medicine avoided the whole area of diet and nutrition?
* Why wasn't there a more integrated approach combining Western medicine with complementary therapies?

I was desperately looking to find answers to these questions. Surely there was some rational explanation? Despite not having the answers, I decided I would pursue the subject in depth. I soon discovered that there was information everywhere I looked, and surprisingly it was not all that incomprehensible or particularly complicated.

I learned that this disease is caused by deficiency and toxicity. Each of us have cancers growing inside of us from time to time. What stops their growth getting out of hand is a healthy immune system. I also learned that, given the correct tools, our own body has the remarkable ability to heal itself, but that if we don't provide our body with the correct building blocks we can seriously impede its function. Symptoms get worse with time and eventually our health will degenerate. The body will fail to protect itself from disease when we do not provide it with the correct nourishment to make healthy cells. So in order to help the body recover and thrive, it is imperative to provide a regular supply of food that is not stripped of its immune-boosting nutrients. Fresh, raw, unprocessed foods provide us with the best essential components for health and are the finest medicine that nature can provide.

I was so determined in my quest to beat the cancer that I immediately set about making some corrective changes. These changes were intended to support myself through the six months of chemotherapy, the 25 radiation treatments, and the operation that now faced me. I was also hoping these changes would insure against future recurrences of the cancer. Whatever the outcome was to be, I was not about to sit around and wait until I got to the point of no return. I had to find a way to help myself.

Initially I realized that these treatments were going to be very debilitating and I worked hard to try to counteract the effects on my immune system. What happened next amazed me! I had never experienced healing to this extent on a physical level before. As I switched to more nourishing foods, I first began to notice the disappearance of the arthritis in my right hand and shoulder that had plagued me for many years. This was really significant for me, as I could see the benefits happening in front of my eyes. I wore reading glasses and I realized I was picking them up less and less. As an added bonus I also lost my middle-aged spread!

I will freely admit that having arthritis and wearing reading glasses are not such major problems when one has been diagnosed with cancer. But my positive attitude and actions were rewarding me with some very positive feedback from my body. So I began to look seriously at the bigger picture. I was hoping to heal myself from cancer and the side-effects of its treatments. Of course I couldn't see the cancer itself, but I could see these welcome and apparent changes to my body. This was confirmation to me that when you give the body what it needs, it will speed recovery and reward you by supporting the natural state of health. I realized then that by boosting the immune system *my body was back in charge*.

I remember thinking to myself: 'If only I had learned all of this information earlier in my life! Why had I waited till my choice was so desperate?' I was truly amazed at the incredible intelligence inherent in the human body … *when* we take care of it.

In this book I will share with you the simple changes I made to support, sustain and improve my health throughout this challenging and difficult time. It appeared that the only option open to me where I could make a difference was with what was going into my shopping basket. After all, I had no time to waste wondering if it was the environment or some other unknown reason that was giving me the cancer. Neither my mother, who lived to the ripe old age of 93, nor either of my sisters had ever developed cancer – surely it could not be hereditary?

It was very frustrating and disappointing to discover that none of my doctors was able to give me the answer to why I had developed this disease for a second time, or indeed why I had developed it in the first place! It still baffles me how so much money has been spent on cancer research and yet the medical profession cannot tell us what the cause is! How can this be? Thankfully, evidence is now available that clearly points to a connection between diet and cancer. This evidence is available from the Bristol Cancer Centres database.

Encouraged by these positive changes to my body and coupled with the strong notion that nutrition was the bottom line when it comes to good health, it seemed a logical and natural step for me to investigate this area and learn how to improve my diet. How difficult could it be to switch to foods which, according to what I was reading, could fight this disease? I will admit that at times I found a lot of the information I got from reading and attending lectures confusing and a minefield of contradictions, nevertheless

I was determined to press ahead. After all, when on holiday don't we experiment with different foods all the time? I also know that for many of us, when we think of health foods we automatically assume they will be tasteless and awful. One reason for this is possibly because we don't know how to prepare them. This was another area where I was keen to learn more. I wanted to find delicious and better ways to prepare food.

From all the lectures I attended and experts I spoke to, the most astounding fact I learned was that when food is cooked or steamed above 43°C (115°F) it destroys almost 100 per cent of the enzymes in these foods. I also discovered that the enzymes destroyed in cooking are vital for breaking down foods into smaller, more usable nutrients, and this in turn helps the body absorb these nutrients from the foods more efficiently. Our health pays a significant price when we eat foods without these enzymes. This was when I realized that there are some foods we eat largely for comfort and others we eat largely for nourishment.

As I learned more and began to prepare these foods, it was natural for me to want to pass this on to my family. Like every wife and mother I wanted to give the best nourishment to my husband and children. Let me assure you this was not met with open arms and there was an argument almost every evening around our kitchen table. Changing eating habits can be very challenging, especially for teenagers and children. This is why adding good foods, rather than eliminating poor ones, can be a better way of proceeding. You don't spend all your time feeling hungry or thinking about the foods you cannot have, and – trust me – as you progress you naturally begin to stop buying expensive, convenience junk foods.

Although not an easy task, in the end I decided to get sneaky and find ways of disguising these nourishing foods and sparing myself the arguments and the opposition. I even managed to make Sunday dinner with gravy that contained millet without them noticing. It may not sound very appetizing, but believe me it certainly passed the test with my bunch. They already suspect that I sneak as many nourishing ingredients as I can get away with into their food, but now that my secret is out it may not be so easy in the future.

Where foods and nourishment are concerned, the evidence is neither black nor white. I often think of the millions that are spent on general education for our children, and yet very little of that time and money is put into educating them on the one thing they must do for the rest of their lives – EAT. Must we wait until scientific evidence proves beyond a shadow of a doubt that poor diet leaves us with a vulnerable immune system which can allow disease to develop?

Some of us may simply not have the luxury of that time and cannot afford to sit around and wait until there is conclusive scientific proof. Waiting until we're ill can sometimes be too little too late. Of course I understand that it is difficult to make large amounts of money from encouraging people to eat fruits and vegetables, and I strongly suspect that the financial motivation does not exist to fund research that proves the simple connection between good foods and health.

One of the most important steps we can make towards better health is to take responsibility for our own nourishment. I know we all have a list of excuses why we can't make juice, drink more water, or prepare some real food, but please don't immediately dismiss these suggestions. Better to make one change than not try at all. *Moderation* is the key to success when making lifestyle changes. The truth is you *can* do it if you *want* to. The choice is yours.

Over the past six years I have seen many people implement these changes into their lives without much difficulty, and believe it or not 80 per cent of these people were already healthy! It is not just cancer patients who are seeking changes to their lifestyles. The changes I made have certainly improved my life beyond measure.

Although frivolous in comparison with cancer, losing my middle-aged spread was a nice bonus for me and I was not about to look a gift horse in the mouth. Recently my daughter Sarah was watching a family video and commented how she could not believe the change in my body shape since I changed my lifestyle. I have also experienced major improvements to my skin and hair, which again is very encouraging.

Throughout my gruelling and arduous cancer treatment, people told me how amazingly strong and courageous I was – though I must confess I felt I had none of these qualities. I had all the normal feelings of anger, resentment and incredible fear. No matter how discouraging or difficult it was to face this punishing and trying time, I simply had no choice other than to get up and get on with it. Determination was the key for me, and by educating and informing myself I found that the knowledge I gained gave me the power to help, first myself, and then many others. I learned to take the good from a situation, and received great satisfaction and fulfilment in watching the people I helped thrive and return to good health. One of these people recently wrote to me the following few lines:

The information I learned from you at the outset of my illness was like a roadmap to good health. It was such a relief to feel empowered and to be an active participant in my own recovery by simply changing some habits. The juicing and water drinking are now automatic routines that apply to the whole family. We have truly shifted our comfort zones and really feel the benefit of our new habits. I am fortunate to have made a full recovery from cancer and I now feel armed with a new confidence about my health and my future. My illness was a wake-up call, and by simply embracing the changes you recommend has given me the energy to focus on the future and has liberated me from the worries of my past history.

Joy

Remember – I am no expert and I understand if you might be sceptical, yet through my classes and lectures I have taught cancer patients (young and old), doctors, nurses, biochemists and many other professionals about my common sense approach of simply passing on the four steps that helped me return to good health.

You can read my full story in my first book, *The Choice*. It is the story of a very ordinary mother's life. From the responses I have received it would seem to provoke many different interpretations for its many readers. The book reflects why and how so many people have come to listen to my simple message and approach – and why I believe nutrition is the bottom line in maintaining health.

The priorities in the recipes in this book are health, taste and simplicity. They have been put together in a pronounced user-friendly way. Together with the chefs from Cornucopia Dublin, we have worked on each recipe's taste and simplicity, and in my opinion we have succeeded in providing recipes to suit all manner of tastes. We will be using familiar foods that reflect today's modern lifestyle and are widely available in supermarkets, though you may also need to make an occasional trip to your healthfoods store!

Here you will learn how to prepare healing therapeutic juices, scrumptious inviting salads, snacks, dips, mouth-watering main meals, and yummy nutritious guilt-free treats to add a little sweetness to your lives. I hope you enjoy the easy preparation and delicious tastes of these wonderful foods that will contribute to a more vibrant and healthier you!

Step One:
Juice Up Your Life!

*I often think we are obsessed with cleaning the outside
of the body, yet we forget about cleaning the inside …*

The Low-down on Juicing

Juices are highly concentrated forms of nutrition and are of particular value to people fighting any kind of disease ... They will revolutionize your body's ability to heal itself and boost your natural defences.

Juicing – A Way of Life

If there was ever a sure-fire way of improving your health and well-being, then it is juicing. Juices are packed with nutrients and bursting with flavours. I immediately felt the benefits of these easy-to-prepare juices, with their delicious taste being an extra advantage. I can promise you there is no better way to recharge your batteries than with freshly extracted fruit and vegetable juices. **Juices have outstanding nutritional qualities and they begin their cleaning and healing of the body within 15 to 30 minutes of being consumed.** Compared with solid foods, juices are easily assimilated by the body. This means the workload on our digestive system is reduced, which facilitates more efficient cleansing and elimination. Our systems are very often overloaded and clogged up with accumulations of wastes and toxins that constantly stream into the body, and green juices such as cucumber and celery are amazing 'spring-cleaners' and an easy way to detox the body. Juices are a perfect means to stimulate better elimination of wastes and toxins, and also assist with the detoxification process.

I often think we are obsessed with cleaning the outside of the body, but we tend to forget the important task of cleaning out the intestines. Believe me, these cleansing drinks will flush out your system very thoroughly, and when taken first thing in the morning they will move mountains! They are also less expensive and far less invasive than other detox methods now available, such as colonic irrigation. I personally have seen many students with long histories of chronic constipation and congested intestines alleviate these conditions with great success by taking green juices.

Juices are highly concentrated forms of nutrition and are of particular value to people fighting any kind of disease. Because of their therapeutic properties and amazing healing powers they are used in many natural healing centres throughout the world. They will revolutionize your body's ability to heal itself and boost your natural self-defences, and you will see and feel the difference.

A dear friend of mine, Ronald, is the best testament for juicing I have ever seen. He juices every day, has the energy of a 20-year-old, attends the gym, travels frequently, takes care of his invalid wife, and also tends his large vegetable garden. He is now 83 years old and is alert, active and productive with the most amazing (hydrated) skin you have ever seen. Why am I so amazed at Ronald's health and vitality? Because most of us have come to believe that ageing is synonymous with disease and infirmity, and that by the time we reach our eighties we ought to have 'one foot in the grave'. Rather than accepting that the inevitable consequence of ageing means physical degeneration and disease, Ronald has taken responsibility for his own well-being. He has taken the matter of ageing healthily into his own hands and is now reaping the rewards of his fruitful diet. *Sláinte!*

Of course it is inevitable that ageing will bring about marked physiological change, but by nurturing your body with the correct fuel you can make a significant contribution to ageing healthily – you can help your body become and continue to be a picture of health, regardless of how old you are.

What better way to increase your intake of fruits and vegetables and, equally important, to increase your children's intake, than with delicious juices? Including these in your diet will be one of the healthiest steps you can take for your body. I have noticed I am at my absolute best when I am drinking these juices. They give you the stamina to live life to the fullest and I guarantee you will see positive results.

With just two glasses of juice per day you can consume large quantities of fruits and vegetables, and the recommended daily amounts can be easily reached. For two 8-ounce glasses of juice per day you will need 6–8 portions of fruits and vegetables, whereas it would take the entire afternoon to chew your way through that many pieces. The point of increasing our intake is to provide our bodies with enough vitamins, minerals, enzymes and trace elements to support a healthy body and give sustained energy levels. **A well-hydrated body is essential for good skin**

and enhanced vitality. If you find drinking large amounts of water difficult, these delicious drinks can easily increase your fluid intake. Juices are also an enjoyable way of increasing fluid levels after a work-out. Your shopping list will change, but you will gradually get a feel for the extra amounts of fruit and vegetable shopping required.

Because these juices are uncooked, they are loaded with enzymes, vitamins, minerals and amino acids. Enzymes are the catalysts for the breakdown of our foods, and I cannot stress their importance highly enough. You will find them mentioned throughout this book. The large amounts of phytonutrients in these juices are amazing for boosting energy levels and good looks. They help maximize our ability to fight disease and boost our capacity for self-healing.

At one point I was juicing large amounts of carrots, as they are rich in carotinoids such as beta-carotene. It was no surprise that I noticed my eyesight improve, as beta-carotene is fantastic at enhancing eyesight. Juices are also a wonderful short-term antidote to a lack of energy or a sluggish metabolism, and you can increase your intake of these vital nutrients without any artificial colourings, flavours or preservatives.

There is unquestionably a new proliferation of juice bars sweeping the country at present. Indeed, in the quest for health we have taken to the juicing habit superbly. The growth in this particular market shows that consumers have definitely become more aware of the connection between diet and health. A rock festival recently attended by my daughter Sarah had queues a mile long at the juice bar. All I can say is 'great' – I am delighted to see young people embracing this change for the better.

One question I am asked repeatedly is if I use organic fruit and vegetables. My reply is always the same: *absolutely*. If you took an apple from a tree in your garden and then sprayed it with a chemical, would you then eat this apple or hand it to your child to eat? I think not. Remember, where there are commercial interests we, the consuming public, are not always given the correct information. Now that the consumer has become better informed and is more aware of the benefits of eating organically-grown produce, it has become much more widely available in the marketplace. There is no doubt that 'eating organic' is definitely catching on and is our only guarantee of purity.

The organic end of the market is now becoming an expanding and lucrative business. You might wonder why. The reason certainly seems to be in direct response to the growing interest and demands of consumers for superior products – superior both in terms of having a better flavour and better nutritional value. Many of the producers now enthusiastically display their certification that will assure you of the authenticity of their organically-grown products. Organic classification ensures that the products are approved and inspected regularly by an independent organization that checks for compliance with all regulations and specifications. With the influx of chemicals into the food chain, exposure to pesticides, insecticides, fungicides, herbicides and chemical fertilizers can now have far-reaching consequences. You should be fully aware of these chemically-laden foods, as you may get a little bit more than you bargained for in your shopping basket.

It is no longer difficult to locate organic foods, but if you are unable to obtain organic produce, peeling off the top layer of skin from the fruit and vegetables you buy will generally remove any surface residues of chemicals. However, peeling is not the ideal solution, as many of the important nutrients in fruit and vegetables are contained directly under the skin.

Along with the benefits of not exposing ourselves to absorbing foods that are irradiated and sprayed with pesticides, there is the added benefit of the sheer taste of these fruits and vegetables. In comparison, the conventionally grown chemically-sprayed varieties with their long sell-by dates are tasteless imitations of the real thing. These foods may essentially look perfect, but don't be fooled as they offer little in the way of true flavour or nourishment.

Does it cost more? Well yes, of course it commands a higher price due to the fact that the growing and harvesting of these crops is much more labour intensive. Although this is not always strictly the case, as I have on occasion bought cheaper organic produce than the chemically sprayed variety. It roughly costs about one-third more to buy organic foods … but it's worth it. What with these harmful chemicals infiltrating our everyday diet, choosing organic foods may be your only option if you don't want to bite off more then you can chew.

With organic juices you are guaranteed freshness and they are so much tastier than packaged concentrates and cordials. Many of these packaged juices are full of sugar and are devoid of enzymes, as they are pasteurized and heat treated. I don't find juicing time-consuming; I think it's more about deciding to do it and then carrying it through. It takes about five minutes to make a juice and five minutes to clean up after, and I consider this time well spent. **Juices are always better consumed within 15 minutes of preparation while the enzymes and nutrients are at their best.** Don't be tempted to make large batches to last for a few days, as oxidation will occur and this will rapidly diminish the nutrients in the juice. Another tip is that if you are going out and you decide to take a juice with you, store it in a stainless-steel vacuum flask with ice to slow down oxidation. This will definitely be better for you than a cup of coffee.

The Right Juicing Equipment

If ever there was a piece of equipment worthy of a place in your kitchen, it has got to be a juicer. It is important to spend a bit of time choosing the correct machine for your needs. There are so many brands on the market today that you could be forgiven for not knowing which one is best. I myself survived for some time with the centrifugal type of juicer, which is of the less expensive variety readily available in the high street. I use the word *survived* because I found it fiddly and difficult juicing daily with this type of machine. The reasons for this were:

* Centrifugal machines are difficult to clean. Be sure to check this out before purchasing a juicer. It is an extremely important point to remember, as cleaning can be time-consuming especially if you're trying to fit making juices into an already full and busy schedule.
* They are wasteful as they produce a lot of pulp, which is not very cost effective.
* They mainly extract the water from the fruit and vegetables. You will notice this as the juice separates after a very short time.
* They can also destroy the nutrients in the juice, as these machines operate at very high speeds (about 3,000 revs per minute).

The juicer I now use is a masticating juicer. I carried out a lot of research on many different machines before I discovered the machine I wanted. (You will find addresses in the Resources section to help you if you wish to purchase a masticating juicer). My trusty juicer will juice anything you throw at it. I have had trouble-free use of this robust machine for the past six years.

Juicing is not the only thing I use this machine for; it has many other uses and I have found it to be an effortless way of making cookies and crackers. I feel sure I haven't yet explored its full potential. Many of my students amaze me when they tell me of the wonderful foods they have managed to make with this machine. **Natural healing centres throughout the world have been using these masticating machines for many years.** They grind and crush the fruits and vegetables slowly, at around 110 revolutions per minute. While masticating juicers are more expensive, I have certainly found my machine to be worth the extra cost. It provides several advantages:

- ❖ The slow grinding process produces a good-quality juice loaded with enzymes and nutrients. Independent studies show that they extract up to 74 per cent more vitamins and minerals than centrifugal juicers.
- ❖ These machines are easy to clean and, believe me, this is a huge advantage and a major selling point of masticating juicers. A quick tip: after a juicing session I open the nozzle at the front of the machine and, with the machine turned on, pour a jug of water through the machine. This cleans out 90 per cent of any leftover waste and there is virtually no cleaning left to do.
- ❖ They produce very little pulp. I collect what little pulp there is in a small glass and pass it through the machine again and again to squeeze more juice from it.
- ❖ Wheatgrass and all leafy green vegetables (major sources of chlorophyll and nutrients) can be easily juiced in these twin-gear masticating juicers. With the cheaper machines these leafy greens get stuck and can jam the machine.

These are just a few of the things to consider when purchasing a juicer, and I hope you find this short analysis of their relative effectiveness useful. I have researched and discussed the merits of various types of juicers with many experts and they all seem to have come to the same or similar conclusions.

Wheatgrass Juice

Wheatgrass juice is a superfood that deserves a mention all of its own. It has become justifiably popular and it is now best-known for helping those with weakened resistance because of its incredible effectiveness at fighting disease. It contains high quantities of minerals and is one of the richest sources of beta-carotene, vitamin C and vitamin B_{17} (a substance that is thought to destroy cancer cells). It is extremely valuable in suppressing bacterial growths and is highly effective at eliminating stored toxins, as it is rich in chlorophyll which aids the body in purifying the liver.

Indeed, wheatgrass is so powerful that 1 ounce of it is said to be the equivalent of over 2 lb of fresh fruit and vegetables in terms of vitamins, minerals, trace elements and phytonutrients. Humans cannot eat wheatgrass. It can only be digested in a juice form, because in this form it can be easily assimilated and the body can utilize its storehouse of nutrients. Juice bars up and down the country are now supplying this wonderfully powerful juice. Indeed, it has become one of the top-selling health foods in the world. *More details on growing your own wheatgrass can be found on pages 67–9.*

Let's Juice

You will notice I have used a lot of apples in the mouth-watering recipes that start on page 119 – mainly because apples are readily available all year round, and the majority of people have apples regularly available in their fruit bowl. Furthermore, apple seeds are a wonderful source of nitrosilides, which can help protect us from disease. Carrots also feature largely in the recipes, as again they are an everyday vegetable which most of us use and they are readily available. The use of readily available fruits and vegetables is important as it can be frustrating not having the fruits and vegetables available when you decide to make a juice. I hope you enjoy the different tastes, as well as the health benefits that juicing will bring to you. Remember; keep it simple and enjoy it!

Yummy-for-your-tummy Smoothies

Enzyme-rich smoothies are another wonderful way to kick-start your day. They are the ultimate fast-food as they can be whipped up in seconds. You simply throw all your favourite ingredients into a blender and whiz them up. What could be more convenient and easy?

I should point out at this stage that juices and smoothies are completely different drinks, although both are beneficial. Smoothies, which include some fibre, require more prolonged digestion. With juicing the cellular walls of the fruit and vegetables are broken down and only the liquid is extracted, leaving the fibre behind. Fibre, which is important for health, can easily be added throughout the day by the intake of other foods. Digesting foods is one of the hardest jobs your body has to undertake, but in these liquid drinks we can digest and assimilate their precious nutrients much more readily.

Smoothies take less time to prepare than the average breakfast of cereal, toast and coffee. Children are especially attracted to their yummy creamy textures and colours. **Nourishing ingredients such as soaked fruits, seeds and nuts can be used as thickeners, and also nourishing essential fats can easily be blended into smoothies.** Smoothies by their nature tend to use more fruits than vegetables, subsequently these will satisfy the sweetest tooth. Remember the old saying, though – *a little of what you fancy does you good* – and try not to overindulge. For sustained energy levels throughout the day, these drinks offer good nourishment for breakfast or lunch.

The majority of households have blenders or even hand-blenders these days, so I hope you will not need to purchase another piece of equipment. If you do have to invest in one you will find them useful for many tasks such as making soups, smoothies, patés and stuffing. Hand-blenders are wonderful, as in the past when I would make soup I'd pour it into the food processor to liquidize the vegetables, and end up spilling most of it on the counter-top or on myself, so needless to say I find the hand-blender a big improvement!

Some of the smoothie recipes included in this book has been given to me by my friends Stephen and David. They run a juice bar in Wicklow called 'The Happy Pear' and all I can tell you is they are absolutely gorgeous … the smoothies, that is, not the happy pair! Thanks for your kind help, lads!

I hope that the smoothie recipes will give you ideas for some quick and healthy starts to your day.

Step Two: Powerful Foods

*Nature intended us to eat growing foods and
living foods that are full of vitality ...*

To Cook? Or Not to Cook?

We have been habitually conditioned to using foods that are stripped of nutrients and leave us with exhausted immune systems. We very often overlook the simple fact that eating raw food is what Mother Nature intended.

This next section looks at the issues of preparing food, and the benefits of eating an uncooked diet. Nature intended us to eat growing foods and living foods that are full of vitality. What nature did not intend was for us to zap the life out of what we eat, resulting in us consuming tasteless, bland, dead food that in no way resembles nourishment. **The result of continually eating highly processed foods is that we become increasingly susceptible to disease as the body loses the ability to repair itself.** On top of this is the added concern that we then attempt to reinstate a sense of taste into these now tasteless foods by overloading them with salt and sugar.

The term 'raw food' can often conjure up an image of something unwelcoming or even unpleasant. For this reason most of the recipes will be referred to as 'uncooked foods'. Any negative connotations of raw food soon disappears when you begin to taste how delicious this food can actually be.

I can fully appreciate how the idea of eating raw cuisine can seem strange and daunting. Many people think that raw food consists of a plateful of 'rabbit food', believing the meal will consist of leaf or two of lettuce and few sticks of carrot! On the contrary, you will find that the dishes included in my recipes will have you drooling in anticipation of their amazing variety of tastes and flavours. Crackers, crisps, pizzas, biscuits and cakes can all be prepared without destroying their nutrients. Using fresh, colourful foods takes the boredom out of food preparation and you will soon find yourself eating food of a far superior quality while also saving yourself some time and money.

This trend is rapidly gaining momentum, although there is most definitely nothing new about the phenomenon. Humans have been eating this way since the beginning of time. What is new about the trend of eating raw food is the method of preparation. Chefs and novices alike have now created new, adventurous recipes for raw foods that are not devoid of nutrients and yet retain the appearance of cooked food. My experience of this dietary awakening first occurred while on holiday with my husband Ger when we visited 'Juliano's' – a raw food restaurant in Santa Monica, California. To this day he still talks about his surprise at the amazing taste of what was a totally uncooked meal. And believe me, this was praise indeed from him, as I am still working (with limited success, I might add) on converting him into a better way of eating. Looking back now, I remember that he was constantly sampling the foods on my plate. It did illustrate to me at that time that the only way to win him over was to learn for myself how to prepare these recipes.

Uncooked and Ready to Eat!

Another fact we often overlook is that eating raw food is what Mother Nature intended. Heating, processing and refining food knocks the life out of it, and I strongly suspect that these practices are conducted more in the interests of the food producers than those of the consumer. Not only are these overcooked foods lacking in nutrients but also of concern is the huge issue of the destruction that occurs in their preparation. **When we heat food above 43°C (115°F) we destroy almost all the enzymes (essential for digestion and breaking up foods into smaller nutrients), nearly all the vitamins, and some of the minerals.** Even steaming food is not as healthy as you might think. The high temperatures that result from steaming mean that, again, you may be destroying the valuable nutrients originally stored inside the food in its raw state.

Enzymes Explained

Uncooked foods have an abundance of enzymes that utilize and assist the process of digestion. A good digestive system supports the body's basic needs and functions, and this leads to better health. You cannot have one without the other. On the contrary, poor digestion leads to malnutrition and toxicity. It is within the digestive system that most of the problems of ill-health occur. **Uncooked foods are much less demanding on our bodies and are digested much faster than the cooked versions of these foods.** Cooked foods, on the other hand, stress the body and trigger its defences, as they are recognized as invaders. When our bodies are constantly working to replace the nutrients destroyed in the cooking process, it has a profound impact on our health. In addition to this, foods that are overheated can produce dangerous free radicals which attack our body tissue and can lead to diseases such as cancer.

On that note, I will provide a quick update on the story of Susie – a wonderful woman I wrote about in my previous book. I have had so many requests for more information on Susie's health that I felt compelled to give her story a second mention. Susie and her husband John sought my help and advice some years back. She had been diagnosed with ovarian cancer which had then spread into her lungs. Over the past few years she underwent three separate six-month sessions of chemotherapy. Then, four years ago, she made the choice to introduce some changes to her diet and lifestyle in order to give her body the food it required. She is now reaping the rewards. She recently told me that she truly believes that her new diet has saved her life. Susie is a wonderful example of a courageous woman who took responsibility for her self-healing. Over the past few years we have become good friends and it has been the best tonic for me to see this lovely woman thrive and return to health. Now she can happily enjoy life with her devoted husband John.

It is important to be aware that nine times out of ten we miss the small truths when reading about nutrition, and very often this turns out to be the most vital information of all. The most important fact we seem to misunderstand, or perhaps are reluctant to confront, is around preparing our food. The convenience of cooking is not always a Godsend for our unfortunate bodies. **A microwave meal may save you 20 minutes of cooking, but by heating foods at high temperatures we destroy the most important nutrients –** *the enzymes.* These busy workers do all of the work in breaking up foods inside the body, and foods without these precious enzymes can place a heavy burden on the digestive system and leave us feeling sleepy and lethargic. With the absence of enzymes in the food we eat, the pancreas is required to work harder to produce them. Consequently it is difficult for the body to function properly. If we consume uncooked foods, we can provide our bodies with the precious stores of enzymes needed to repair and heal itself efficiently.

It is not left unnoticed by the body when we use unnatural cooking methods. Nature finds a way of fighting back and the process of accelerated ageing occurs, as dead food cannot rejuvenate or regenerate the cells of the body. Many experts believe that enzyme deficiencies are the root cause behind every degenerative disease. You may think that you are getting the necessary nutrients in your food by checking what it says on the label or packaging, but if foods are not properly *assimilated* their nutritional content is of little use to the body. The facts are clear: when we destroy these indispensable working enzymes the value of the food we consume is greatly diminished. Many of the illnesses and complaints we have come to accept today could be avoided by incorporating nourishing foods containing these vital enzymes into our diets. We can then properly assimilate and absorb the nutrients from the foods we choose to eat. One thing is for certain – integrating these foods into your diet will help improve your overall health.

Dehydrated Foods

Uncooked foods are often prepared in dehydrators because they warm the foods slightly without destroying the nutrients, and give the finished dish the appearance of being cooked. These machines are inexpensive (see the Resources section for more details) and you can produce satisfying, tasty and enzyme-rich foods for yourself and your family. Dehydrators intensify the flavours of foods by extracting the water from them; this will also intensify the flavours of the foods. Dehydrators are also an efficient way of drying fruits such as apples, pineapples, mango and bananas. You can also easily prepare your own sun-dried tomatoes. You simply slice the fruits, dip them in some lemon juice to stop discolouration, and place them in the dehydrator. These healthy snacks make wonderful little treats, especially for lunch boxes.

Apart from learning to dehydrate (which is a relatively simple process), you do not need many culinary skills to prepare an uncooked meal. Maybe the concept of dehydrated food is totally new to you, and because we have eaten cooked foods for most of our lives, there is always a transition period. Dehydrated foods are excellent at bridging this gap. The key is to add a new dish on one or two days a week, allowing your taste buds to adjust to the new flavours. Even a small bit of restructuring like this will mean you are far more likely to succeed with the changes in the long term. It is definitely worth making the effort to enjoy these delicious natural tastes that will provide your body with much more nutrition.

Dehydrators

A dehydrator is an inexpensive piece of equipment that won't take up much space in your kitchen. This useful machine can greatly increase your ability to prepare delicious foods that are not depleted of vital nutrients essential for a healthy strong body for yourself and your family. Dehydrating food can take time, although the time is not usually spent in the actual preparation of the food, but rather in the length of time required for drying out the food. Unlike an oven, it is not necessary to watch the dehydrator constantly as there is no risk of burning the food. You simply check on it occasionally until the food is ready to eat.

Drying sheets (Teflex sheets) are often used in dehydrating foods; they look similar to parchment paper but are reusable and inexpensive.

Cooked but Nutritious …

While uncooked foods are without any doubt more nutritious, this doesn't mean that it is always harmful to include some cooked meals in your diet. Warm, cooked dishes will provide you with some well-deserved comfort so often necessary at the end of a hard day. Being creative with food can stop you becoming uninterested in or fed up with the foods you eat. So don't be afraid to experiment! Getting children to pitch in (and yes, I do know this option can be messy!) can be a sure way to get them eating healthily. They always feel proud of what they have made themselves.

The cooking process will of course take away some of the nutrients in the food, so make sure to choose some dishes from the uncooked recipes to ensure you get good amounts of nutrients throughout the day. With the clever addition of garlic, sprouts, sprouted grains and seaweeds at the end of the cooking process you can also add some valuable nutrients back into these dishes. Cooked foods require very little chewing and slip down the throat easily. I find when I eat cooked foods I still feel quite hungry afterwards. This may be the reason why so many people feel the need for desserts and coffees after their meals.

Uncooked foods require a lot of chewing, and when we chew foods properly our hunger is more satisfied. Chewing properly also helps pre-digest food. When the foods are mixed with saliva this starts the breakdown and digestion of the food, especially of carbohydrates. Chewing also helps increase their absorption.

Recipes are only general guidelines and ideas – they are by no means written in stone, and it is worthwhile experimenting with some of your own ideas. Presentation is always important as it makes the food appealing – throwing it all onto a plate, even if you are busy and hurried, does not always work as the food may then end up in the bin. Be sure to adjust the seasonings to suit your own tastes. I rarely use salt myself, but for the family I use very small amounts to ensure they eat and enjoy the dishes prepared. Good seasoning will make the blandest ingredients taste better, so I strongly suggest you try to get used to using herbs and spices. I tend to use turmeric quite a lot in my recipes. I find it is wonderful for adding colour to your dishes and it also has many healing qualities.

For the past five years I have eaten vegetarian foods. Before you ask – no, I am definitely not going to preach to you about giving up meat, fish, or chicken. You may well decide to add these meats to some of the recipes that I have provided. But let me assure you that there is nothing lacking or depriving about living a vegetarian lifestyle. Indeed, nowadays I often find that when I am eating with my family and friends they are often more interested in the foods on my plate than in what they are eating themselves! This may be because the foods I choose to eat look so fresh, colourful and delicious.

One of the leading causes of ill-health in today's modern society is the over-consumption of meat products. The risks are all too obvious – we read every day about the transmission of infections and viruses that infiltrate our food chain. I did not set out to become a vegetarian, in hindsight it actually developed as a natural reaction when I began to learn about the negative effects that animal products could have on our health. My mother often told me about the shortages of meat during the Second World War and of how she ate mostly vegetarian food during that period. When I investigated this era I discovered there was a dramatic decrease in diet-related diseases, such as heart disease, at this time.

Every book I've read spoke of the low incidence of degenerative diseases (such as heart disease and cancer) among vegetarians, and of the many cancer-preventing phytochemicals that are available in plant foods. The grim prospects of the increased risk of disease with the intake of animal products finally made up my mind, and as I was prepared to leave no stone unturned, and it was a matter of some urgency for me, I decided to give vegetarianism a go.

Personally I believe that my decision to eat only vegetarian foods has freed me from the dangers of many of the diseases that are prevalent in today's animal products, such as BSE and salmonella. My personal motivation towards vegetarianism was definitely for health reasons. But whether your interest in eating this way stems from a desire to rejuvenate the body, protecting animal rights, or perhaps protecting the environment, vegetarianism has without a doubt a lot to offer and many wonderful benefits. Contrary to popular belief, I have observed that the many people I have come to know who live a vegetarian lifestyle have enormous energy and an exceptional glow about them. Indeed, many of them have a deep social conscience and are especially aware of the environment.

The biggest question you are asked continually when you become a vegetarian is 'How do you get your proteins?' The answer is quite simple. **Meat is *not* the only source of protein available to us.** Nature has provided us with all the protein we could possibly need. Vegetable protein is available in an abundance of foods such as beans, nuts, seeds and lentils. A very valuable source of protein for any vegetarian should be the grain quinoa. This is especially rich in amino acids (which are proteins broken down into smaller usable nutrients), and yet it is rarely used in contemporary cooking.

One of the biggest problems facing vegetarians today is the fact that the majority of their food is cooked. Remember, real health cannot be sustained on a diet which consists primarily of mostly cooked and processed foods, as this is largely due to the fact that the molecular structures of foods are greatly disrupted by the process of cooking. Yes, of course, cooked foods do retain some vitamins, minerals, fats, proteins and carbohydrates. However, the process of cooking, frying, sautéing, boiling and micro-waving foods greatly alters their nutrient content, and the finished product is nowhere even close to what nature intended us to eat. And so, while we can see that a vegetarian lifestyle offers many benefits which improve human health, it is also apparent that a major problem lies in how we choose to prepare our meals.

I mentioned losing my middle-aged spread earlier on in this book, and how this is an added bonus of eating good food. But let me now put it to you this way: I am now in my fifties and at long last the struggle of having a flat stomach and being able to fit into the jeans I always wanted to wear has become a reality. I now have the figure I wanted for most of my life and there has been no dieting, no guilt, and most definitely *no going without*. For as long as I can remember I spent my life trying to squeeze, shove and pull my way into jeans, skirts, trousers – you name it. It was not that I was greatly overweight, but I certainly had a few extra pounds here and there that I was always trying to lose.

Since I switched to nutritious uncooked foods I visibly lost fat from underneath my chin, from my upper arms, and all round my middle. I didn't actually drop in weight, it was just that it became better spread on my body. This was a great change from all the other times that I tried various fad-diets where I somehow managed to lose weight off all the places I didn't want to! My husband Ger told me it was like being with a 20-year-old again, although I must admit I am not sure how far down the bottle of wine he was when he said that!

All kidding aside, many of my students have had exactly the same response to eating a more uncooked and nutritious diet. One of the best strategies you can employ if you feel you are overweight is to train your eating habits and to put more uncooked foods into your diet. In my experience most people find that making changes to the foods they eat is quite challenging, but if you feel positive about these changes you will find them easier to incorporate into your lifestyle. I have all too often seen people with a various range of problems protest that they cannot possibly change their diet. This is because we no longer use foods rationally to nourish our bodies, instead it has become an emotional crutch. At the same time I do not agree with 'diets', as overly restrictive regimes are difficult to maintain and simply do not work. In fact, they only serve to make you feel deprived and hard done by.

When I teach or speak about health, the biggest problem seems to be the lack of time we have to prepare real food. By the time we get to the end of a busy day, we have neither the time, the inclination nor the energy for preparing food. While I realize that spending time preparing a meal may not always be feasible, and I empathize with these problems, I am also fully aware of the fact that you must work within the boundaries of your family and your work. So I am definitely not suggesting you slavishly follow complicated recipes when your time is tight. Rather, I want to highlight that there are some basic issues to be considered.

Taking the time to prepare proper nutritious food gives you the available energy necessary to sustain your body throughout the day. Some of these recipes are quick to prepare, and the dehydrated foods can be prepared on days off work or Sundays when you can get the kids involved. Julie and I often spend Sundays preparing crisps, cookies, pancakes, crackers and patés for the week ahead.

In order to maintain good energy levels, we need to eat the *correct fuel* for our bodies. This should come from complex carbohydrates, rather than the quick-fix (sugary food) substitutes that are so readily available. We have all become carbohydrate junkies. We do not need what I refer to as 'quick-fix carbohydrates' to give us energy, and more importantly they will not sustain energy levels. I ask you – how often have you eaten junk food and later regretted it because it made you feel so bad? Not only does it make you feel bloated, sleepy and generally unhealthy, but if these sugary deposits are not used up as energy they become stored as fat. On the upside we have become much more aware that it is this excessive intake of carbohydrates which make us fat, and has led to an explosion of low-carb products on the market. We now know beyond a shadow of a doubt that it is not fats that are the main cause of weight-gain and obesity. Dr Atkins has proved this to the masses with his highly controversial minimal-carb/high-protein diet. While I am not in favour of such high-protein diets, there is a lot to be said for bringing about a reduction in refined carbohydrates into our daily eating patterns.

These refined foods clog up the intestinal walls and interfere with nutrient transfer in the body. They also make the body work overtime to metabolize and break them down. Processed cooked foods cannot pass through the gut easily, as the human gut is a complex winding path full of crevasses and pouches. This path is easily blocked unless it is swept through daily with foods rich in enzymes and fibre. As the walls of the colon begin to back up with undigested waste, the stools become hard and difficult to eliminate.

This of course is only the half of the problem … because refined carbohydrates are stripped of adequate amounts of nutrients, our unsuspecting bodies become both over-fed and undernourished.

Nourishment and nutrition are your best options for improving your state of health. For this reason it looks to me like eating good food and changing our thinking towards food are the *only* ways to achieve optimal health.

The Good, the Bad, and the Ugly

I know this is not exactly music to your ears, and it is undoubtedly hard to accept, but when we eat these foods we are slowly digging our own grave. Be warned, if you are a fast-food, dairy-loving sugar addict ... you are not going to like some of the next few pages ...

I said earlier that I prefer to concentrate on the foods we *can* eat rather than the foods we *can't*. The good news is that it is easy to put these powerful disease-fighting foods back into your diet. The process of eating healthily need not be complicated, and in fact as I have said, the secret is to keep it simple – this way you are far more likely to succeed. You can then comfort and nourish the body with delightful scrumptious foods. As I have said repeatedly, foods are the body's major source of nutrients, so enriching a deficient diet will help optimize health and reverse many of the symptoms of disease. If we don't obtain these essential nutrients from our foods, in time the body falls apart. The Good Foods described in this chapter will help you support the body's basic needs and functions. The Bad and the Ugly sections look at the problems associated with sugar, dairy and the wrong fats.

I have always found it better to find alternatives and add them to the diet before eliminating those foods you are already used to. As you will see, the list of good foods that are full of nourishment and vitality are boundless. However, as many of the foods we eat not only lack nourishment but also contain harmful ingredients, I have three groups of foods that I no longer eat.

First I want to make it clear that I am not trying to tell you to 'get with the programme' or preach to you in any way. I have taught enough people to know that if you don't want to change your eating habits then it simply will not happen. I am merely trying to present to you some brief information as I found it. Be warned, if you are a fast-food, dairy-loving sugar addict you are not going to like some of the next few pages. But whatever you decide to include in your diet, please make sure you consider the following:

❖ Don't allow the life-zapping effects of a malnourished diet to leave you with a compromised immune system.
❖ Learn not to be duped by advertising campaigns that will try to turn your head.
❖ Last but not least, don't wait until you get a wake-up call.

The Good ...

I've got the Power

Essential Fats

Essential fats are powerful healing foods that play a complex role in the maintenance of health in the human body. Although many people take essential fats in the form of a supplement, it is actually a food because its source is from green leafy vegetables, seeds, sprouts, cold-water fish, etc. These good fats are better known as omega 3 and omega 6 fats. Essential fatty acids are *not* produced by the body and must come from foods. As our bodies cannot survive properly without these good fats, it is absolutely necessary to introduce a direct food source of these fats into the diet. These fats feed every cell, organ, tissue and gland within the body and are vital for growth and development. As the brain is one of the body's major organs it requires a regular supply of these essential fats for neurological development. Personally, one of the biggest improvements I noticed from using these fats was my mental clarity. Before I introduced these fats to my diet my memory was not quite firing on all cylinders!

Fats make foods tasty, which is one reason why fried food is in such demand. On the opposite side, low-fat ('diet') foods can often taste like cardboard because they lack the necessary fats for taste. The majority of the population nowadays try to avoid fats and are therefore deficient in these essential fatty acids. They are among the most neglected foods in our diet and this is mostly because of the trends towards low-fat diets. **So keep note that good fats keep us slim, and let me emphasize this point as** clearly as I can – *Essential fats do not make you fat. Excessive carbohydrates make you fat.*

If you restrict your carbohydrate intake to what you burn, you will not gain weight. Essential fats help maintain healthy weight levels and can improve a sluggish metabolism. They noticeably increase metabolic rate and energy levels, which in turn help you burn more calories. They increase energy production by helping the body obtain more oxygen, and when we increase energy levels we feel much more active. For this reason essential fats should not be taken at bedtime because they increase energy levels. Essential fats also help to reduce and satisfy cravings, which are often the result of not receiving the proper nutrients through our foods. These fats elevate mood and lift depression, which are among the main reasons why people over-indulge in junk foods smothered in bad fats.

Some of the major advantages of essential fatty acids are:

❖ They lubricate joints and help prevent arthritis by greatly assisting in reducing inflammation and improving mobility in the joints, thereby reducing pain and discomfort.
❖ They balance hormones and reduce the symptoms of PMT and menopause. Many of my friends and students have had excellent results with these problems by increasing their intake of essential fats.
❖ They help protect us from heart attacks and strokes by making blood platelets less sticky, thereby decreasing the likelihood of clot-formation in the arteries.

❖ They are required for the formation of sex hormones and sperm formation.

❖ They protect our immune system and save our DNA (genetic material) from damage.

❖ They significantly help children suffering from dyslexia, hyperactivity and attention deficit disorder.

Last but not least, these fats are nature's moisturizers and play an important role in creating soft, velvety skin. They are nature's best internal cosmetic as they oil the skin from within. Good fats form a barrier against loss of moisture and dehydration, and so dry skin conditions are one of the first signs of a lack of essential fats. As dry skin is not life-threatening, the body will rob from the skin to supply the vital inner organs. You can obtain excellent results with essential fatty acids if you suffer from eczema, acne, psoriasis and other skin conditions. You will also find that your skin will tan better and burn less (another shot at your vanity – but hey, those points tend to hit home!).

Sources of Essential Fats

One of the best sources of essential fats is found in cold-pressed, unrefined oils. This is the only process that will produce top-grade oils that are beneficial to health. Unrefined oils are also full of flavour, and some of them have a rich nutty taste. These good fats are abundant in seed oils such as flax, sunflower and sesame. They are also present in cold-water oily fish, but as most fish harbour parasites and sometimes even environmental poisons, some less desirable substances might accompany the healthy fats in fish. Seed oils are a wonderful source of good fats. They should be refrigerated and stored in dark glass bottles as they are prone to damage from light, heat and oxygen – if subjected to these conditions they will become completely ineffective. These healing fats can be found in the refrigerated section of quality healthfood stores. The correct ratio of fat in your diet is an important factor, as it is necessary to consume double the amount of omega 3 as omega 6. You can add these oils to food (this way your body will absorb them more easily) by adding them to salad dressings, mashed potatoes or steamed vegetables. Start with small amounts, then gradually increasing your uptake to allow your body to adjust.

A List from Nature

One of the biggest requests I have received from my previous book was a list of the foods that I eat. Some of the following foods I eat regularly because they are rich in vitamin B_{17} (beta-cyanophoric glycosides) or the generic term nitrilosides. Nitrilosides are food compounds said to destroy cancer cells selectively. They are described as an anti-neoplastic vitamin (a vitamin that prevents or inhibits the growth and development of malignant cells). Studies show that nitrilosides are highly effective in protecting us from disease (*Journal of Applied Nutrition*, 1970). These foods have been called the 'missing link' in today's diet. Our ancestors ate copious amounts of these foods in their daily diet, but today these foods are almost totally absent from our diets. Fortunately nature has provided us with many common foods which contained these nitrilosides. They are found in the seed kernels of apricots, apple seeds, pear seeds, bitter almonds, walnuts, pecans, blackberries, gooseberries, cranberries, lentils, sprouts and in great abundance in a variety of vegetables. Wheatgrass millet and buckwheat are also good sources of B_{17}. I myself use large amounts of sprouted seeds and grains in my diet to keep it varied.

The Humble Grain

Throughout the history of mankind, cereals have undoubtedly had a major effect on our diets. Grains were once so prized they were often used as currency. To this day many of these grains still remain an important staple food in Asia and Africa. For example, millet is rich in nitrilosides, and this grain was used in bread-making before the Industrial Revolution.

Around the beginning of the last century, millet was replaced with wheat when it was discovered that wheat was an easier grain to grow and was also much cheaper to produce. This simple agricultural change took this important source of vitamin B_{17} away from the population.

The diet of the Hunzas, an ancient tribe who inhabit the foothills of the Himalayas, has been studied because of their lack of disease and their amazing longevity. This community of people consume a variety of foods rich in B_{17} and have aroused interest because they do not suffer from the degenerative diseases that plague the people of the Western world. They use an abundance of millet in soups, cereals and for making dense wholegrain chapatti bread.

Millet

This grain is extremely nutritious and is a staple grain used by one-third of the world's population in China, Japan, Egypt, Africa and India. Research on the nutritional value of millet is still in its infancy, but the results to date are promising. **Millet is easy to digest and is a useful grain for people with coeliac disease as it is gluten-free. It is beneficial for helping eliminate fungal growths and is also rich in iron, magnesium, phosphorus, potassium and B vitamins.** I use this tasty grain as a thickening agent in sauces, soups, stews and gravies as it has a rich flavour.

Buckwheat

Because of its name, buckwheat is often associated with wheat but it is actually a member of the rhubarb family. **Buckwheat contains all eight amino acids, which means that it is a** complete protein. It is also useful for the treatment of high blood pressure because of its rutin content. Rutin is an antioxidant and anti-carcinogen (anti-cancer-causing agent).

Quinoa

This distant relation of the spinach family is renowned for its protein content. When quinoa grains are sprouted they become much more digestible. Quinoa is an excellent source of minerals such as zinc, calcium, iron and magnesium, and it is also gluten-free. I usually add sprouted quinoa to casseroles, stews and soups at the end of the cooking.

Spelt

Spelt is another ancient grain that was cultivated because of its nutritional content. It is easily digested and is a good substitute for wheat flour in bread. Like wheat, it contains gluten, but even those with coeliac disease can tolerate spelt in small amounts.

Super Sprouts

I began sprouting over 15 years ago – and I have to admit I was never very successful at it at first. But even that far back in my life I must have realized there were many benefits to be gained from these wonderful foods. I think the problem I had was that I found the instructions for growing my own laborious and time-consuming, and try as I might I never managed to get it right.

Now at long last I have learned how to cut through all the complicated jargon and keep this process simple and user-friendly. It roughly takes me about five minutes a day to produce a constant supply of these amazing nutritious living foods. Fresh vegetables are also extremely nourishing, but we sometimes forget the word *fresh*. Can we honestly believe that the two-week-old wrinkled specimens in the bottom of our fridge are still going to nourish our bodies? Healing centres, such as Hippocrates in Florida, use sprouts as part of their programme for treating all kinds of diseases, such as cancer, heart disease and arthritis. This is because of their amazing healing powers and anti-cancer properties. These incredible sprouts contain the most concentrated natural source of enzymes, vitamins, minerals and amino acids vital for health. After all, these little seedlings have stored within them the nourishment to support a fully-grown plant.

Learning how to produce a regular supply of organic sprouts can be a wonderful boost to your diet, especially when you consider the dangers of the influx of toxic chemicals into our foods. **Sprouts are living foods. They are constantly growing, right up until the time of consumption. By growing your own you are literally growing your own organic vegetables!** And no – there is no need to become an avid gardener in order to grow sprouts. In fact, with the exception of wheatgrass, you don't even need any soil to grow these powerful healing foods.

You can grow and harvest a good crop of sprouts from just 3 to 4 ounces of seeds. This amount of seeds will produce about 5 litres of sprouts, and the whole process initially takes about three to four days. When you activate the seeds and grains with moisture, their dormant enzymes spring to life and produce a huge amount of life force. When this massive enzyme-release occurs, they begin to grow and soon start to release vitamin C. This process continues for about seven days. They then release a flood of vitamins (including vitamins A, B-complex, C, D and E) and they are also packed full of proteins, enzymes, iron, potassium, magnesium, calcium, amino acids and essential fatty acids.

Sprouts are extremely cheap to produce and are great value for money when you consider their many benefits. They improve the immune system, help the body to flush out waste, and also protect us against disease. Children often grow sprouts in school because they are ready to eat in a short timeframe. If however you don't have the time or can't be bothered to try to give it a go, they can also be purchased in many stores, supermarkets and healthfood stores.

Their visual appeal is a wonderful boost to any salad or sandwich. I usually add them to cereals, soups, stews and sandwiches. Many sprouts do not have distinctive tastes, and because of this you can easily sneak them into meals without the fussy eaters even knowing! Try my delicious omega-rich sprouted sandwich (see page 199). This is a real favourite with my students.

Let's Sprout!

Sprouts can easily be grown in your kitchen. I find there is no need to put them in the dark as they grow very well placed beside your sink. This is a good place to keep them as you are not as likely to forget to rinse them each day. You can grow them in trays that you can obtain from a healthfood store, or my personal preference is to grow them in wide-necked glass jars covered with net or muslin, and secured with an elastic band. Large selections of organic seeds are available from healthfood stores (not from garden centres!). Don't make it complicated; keep the process simple – this way you're more likely to continue sprouting.

- ❖ Soak the seeds in their jars in water overnight or for 6–12 hours.
- ❖ Rinse and drain. They should be placed at a 45-degree angle so the water drains off.
- ❖ Rinse and drain the sprouts twice daily.
- ❖ After a day or two small shoots will appear.
- ❖ Group A can be eaten at this stage (see table on next page).
- ❖ Group B should be allowed to green up for a further 48 hours.
- ❖ They are now ready to eat. Put a lid on the jar and refrigerate the sprouts.

❖ They can be stored for up to a week, but if they have not sprouted, or you forget to rinse them, throw them out and start again.

The following pages contain lists of the easiest variety of sprouts to grow. **The secret of sprouting successfully is to remember to rinse your sprouts twice daily.**

Group A Sprouts
Mung beans

Lentils (whole)

Fenugreek

Chick peas

Sesame seeds

Sunflower seeds

Pumpkin seeds

Millet

Quinoa

❖ These sprouts should be soaked in water for at least 12 (or up to 24) hours.
❖ After 48 hours sprouting should occur.
❖ No greening is necessary with Group A sprouts.

Group B Sprouts

Alfalfa

Broccoli

Garlic

Onion

Red clover

Sandwich boosters

Spicy mixers

❖ These sprouts should be soaked in water for at least 6 (or up to 12) hours.

❖ After 3 days sprouting should occur.

❖ These sprouts should not be left in direct sunlight.

❖ After 2–3 days two leaves should begin to show. These should be allowed to green up for a further 1–2 days.

Grow Your Own Wheatgrass

Although the task of growing your own wheatgrass may seem a bit daunting at first, I can assure you that this is a relatively simple process, and is well worth the effort when you consider the astounding benefits wheatgrass provides. I use wheatgrass in one of my juice recipes as it contributes to making a particularly powerful and healthy juice drink.

It takes about 10 days in all to complete the growing process of wheatgrass, but as I've said – it is well worth the effort. Because of its name, many people believe they cannot actually drink wheatgrass if they are intolerant to wheat, but this is most definitely not the case. When sprouted the gluten in the grain is broken down and the juice is easily assimilated by the body. **When adding wheatgrass to a juice, as I regularly do, remember that it is always best to consume it within 30 minutes of preparation. This is when the nutrients are at their best and can be utilized to strengthen and stimulate the body's healing powers.**

To grow wheatgrass you will need the following:

- 1 cup of winter wheat berries
- 1 14-inch seed tray with holes (available from garden centres)
- 1 small bag of organic soil (available from garden centres)
- 1 spray bottle of water (for misting the seeds)

Growing Wheatgrass

Here's the method of preparation for growing your own wheatgrass:

- Soak 1 cup of wheat berries overnight.
- Fill a tray three-quarters full with soil and mist it with water.
- Spread the soaked berries evenly over the soil.
- Cover and place the tray in the dark for two days.
- Mist the tray with water twice daily.
- After about 2 to 3 days the wheatgrass should begin to appear.
- Now you can place the tray in indirect sunlight.

- ❖ Continue growing for a further six days, watering twice daily, until the grass reaches approximately 7 to 10 inches in height.
- ❖ The wheatgrass is now ready to be used for juicing.
- ❖ Cut the wheatgrass off with a knife close to the soil and gradually feed the grass into the juicer.

See page 133 for the full recipe for wheatgrass juice.

The Bad …

It's Sweet to Be Sugar Free

So you have a sweet tooth – well, you're not alone. Now I don't want to send you into a panic with the thought of giving up your treats. I know I felt it was a bridge too far and it took me quite a bit of time to phase out the sugary treats that I loved to indulge in. But eventually I lost my sweet tooth – believe me, it can be done.

Sugars are one of the most addictive foods in today's diet. I remember when I began to learn the dangers of these foods, for a time I did not really want to take it on board as I couldn't bear the thought of going without my 'fix'. But eventually I managed to move my comfort zone, and I can tell you I definitely feel the enormous benefits of this move. Large amounts of sugars are found in cakes, muffins, biscuits, chocolate and even in white bread and pasta. These are just a few of the sugar-laced foods to which we have become totally addicted. This is probably not exactly music to your ears, and it is undoubtedly hard to accept the fact that when we eat these foods we are slowly digging our own grave. The phrase 'It was to die for' may need a bit of a rethink.

What is it that makes sugar so bad? Apart from rotting your teeth, surely sugar is not *all* that bad for you? Well … I'm afraid it is – and there is no easy way to say it. Sugar is strong enough to penetrate through tooth enamel, so you can only imagine the damage it can cause within your body. When we eat sugary foods they are absorbed much too quickly into the bloodstream and our bodies are pushed into a state of emergency.

Refined sugars have been connected to a host of diseases, including diabetes, cancer, arthritis, heart disease, Crohn's disease and obesity. Because sugar is a refined food it lacks all the nutrients necessary for its digestion and it draws from our bodies stores of enzymes. Natural plant sources of sweeteners like Stevia (liquorice plant) and Agave syrup (cactus plant) can be used instead of refined sugars and are available in good healthfood stores, or small amounts of honey could also be used.

The Highs and the Lows

Every time we eat sugary foods, they cause major imbalances in our bodies. Our unfortunate body systems are then faced with the challenge of trying to restore a state of equilibrium. Yet we delude ourselves that we need something sweet to stop the constant roller-coaster of high and low blood sugar levels. Nothing could be further from the truth. The energy we obtain from sugary foods is short-lived and causes a fast rise in blood sugar levels, usually followed by an abrupt slump. This constant yo-yoing between high and low blood sugar dooms us to a never-ending cycle of short-lived energy. Does this sound familiar? Far from maintaining our sugar levels, this only results in leaving us worn out, burned out and exhausted.

So let's get down to the nitty-gritty. I think it would be fair to say that going without 'your fix' would not make you a happy camper. In fact, you might feel as if you were desperately hard done by. I have used the word 'feel' because it is clear that much of our indulging in these mood-foods are strongly linked to cleverly designed advertising. I believe that we have become brainwashed by the powers of big business.

Remember, large profits are made from getting you hooked on eating more and more of these foods. We have been almost hypnotized into believing in skilful adverts for instant tempting, sexy products. These carefully crafted advertisements aim to make us surrender to their melt-in-the-mouth products regardless of the consequences to our health. Our children are programmed from the earliest age that they can eat these products to their hearts' desire so long as they brush their teeth afterwards. The powers of persuasion have them completely under their spell and lure them in daily with their shamelessly aimed products, and also with the smart placement of these products in shops and supermarkets. Be well on your guard with these refined sugary foods, as they are bound to leave their mark on your health.

Now I do realize I am up against some very stiff competition when I try to convince you to avoid sweet temptations. I would like to encourage you to avoid or at least cut down on these foods. But how on earth are you expected to break free of something that gives you so much pleasure?

The best practical step to succeed with giving up your 'loving relationship' with these foods is to allow yourself one treat per day or a weekend treat. This will ease the way forward and help you eventually phase out the treats without facing the prospect of never eating sugar again. Try my Lovely Love Bites (page 221). They are easy to prepare and will help you with the sugar blues. I make these for Ger, who is an absolute chocoholic. You may well decide to kick the habit straight away, but before you even begin to contemplate giving sugary foods up, be prepared that you will need to make a few decisions. No matter how bad these foods are for you, you will never succeed in giving them up unless you change your way of thinking. Change your thinking and you will be well on your way to losing your fat, your guilt and your sugar blues.

That's *Dairy Bad* for You …

'Them bones them bones need calcium …'

Yes, it is certainly true that our bones need calcium – but contrary to popular belief we do *not* need the calcium we obtain from cow's milk. Consumption of cow's milk maybe a controversial subject, but evidence suggests that it is a dubious source of calcium. Let me first explain that a deficiency in calcium is not the cause of osteoporosis (bone-mass loss and demineralization). It is firstly a disease of excess proteins that increase excess acid in the body. This acid increases the excretion rates of precious calcium and leeches it from our bones.

Yes, I know it may be difficult to grasp that cow's milk is not meant for human consumption when we have been conditioned to believe otherwise for so long. But the fact it is in no way essential to human health. Basically, the human body does not require milk after weaning, as at this stage we produce less of the lactase enzymes necessary for its digestion. Its nutrient profile is completely different to mother's milk. Lactose is a disaccharide that must be broken down in the small intestine by lactase enzymes; if it is not properly absorbed it ferments in the digestive system and is the cause of many digestive problems. Many people have negative responses and are now allergic or lactose-intolerant (lactose is the predominant sugar in milk). To obtain more information about this subject, information is available from www.netdoctor.co.uk/facts/lactoseintolerance.htm.

Lactose intolerance can be responsible for sparking off and producing widespread sensitivities and allergic reactions for those of us who have lost the ability to break down these sugars.

Initially this may be identified as digestive upsets and diarrhoea, then eventually causing inflammation in the mucous membranes and lungs. The sticky mucus produced by consuming dairy products needs to be excluded for a variety of reasons, but mainly because of its effects on the arteries. This outpouring of mucus causes ear infections, runny noses and persistent sore throats. These are recognized as some of the clear allergic reactions that are accentuated and triggered by dairy products. **Most of us recognize if we have a negative response to specific foods, so it is important to go with your instincts in these cases.**

Also escaping our attention is the large concentrations of chemical residues found in milk, cheese and cream. Antibiotic and anti-parasitic drugs are used to eradicate bovine leukaemia viruses and a plethora of other diseases (that I won't even begin to go into) [EU Directive 70/524 February 1999]. As if this were not bad enough, when coupled with the fertilizers and pesticides used in animal feed, this biochemical solution is nothing short of a chemical soup. It may be wise to consider a reduction in dairy products to reduce your exposure to these chemicals.

It may interest you to know that the Chinese – who have a very low incidence of breast and prostate cancers – don't consume dairy products. Professor Jane Plant, one of Britain's most distinguished scientists, developed breast cancer in 1987 and within four years had four recurrences of the disease. Having been given three months to live, she dumbfounded all the experts when she eliminated all dairy products from her diet and experienced the disappearance of the cancer. She has since remained cancer-free for over 12 years. The evidence is pretty compelling when we address the fact that the Chinese also have the lowest rates of osteoporosis in the world.

'Drink up your milk' my mother told me when I was a child. And I did exactly the same to my own children, for many years, in the belief that I was giving them the best nourishment and helping them build strong bones. Now, thankfully, milk is a thing of the past for me. Since I removed almost all dairy from my diet six years ago the benefits have proved very convincing to me. On the rare occasions that I do catch a cold or sore throat, I am no longer affected by congestion from mucus-forming substances. I have also noticed that my youngest daughter Julie no longer suffers from coughing if she catches a cold. A severe or irritating cough can be very distressing, and a reduction in the consumption of dairy products can greatly ease these infections.

It can of course be difficult to give up what we have become accustomed to for most of our lives, and I know that many of my own friends absolutely love cheese. But I doubt that we can continue to ignore that over-consumption of these products will have consequences for our health.

You can certainly substitute and change to the many alternative milks available, or try making your own coconut or almond milk from the simple recipes on pages 151–2. You will find rice milk, oat milk and almond milk much easier to digest, especially for those who are intolerant or sensitive to dairy foods. If cheese is your thing, try my Health Nut's Cream Cheese (page 174). With the exception of small amounts of butter you will notice that I have used no dairy products in the Recipes chapter.

The Ugly ...

'If You Can't Stand the Heat ...'

I have used the word 'ugly' in this section for the simple reason that most heated fats have a horrific impact on our health. Again this may seem over the top, but **when we heat fats they can turn from healing fats into killing fats.** Over the past 30 years fats have developed a very bad name, so much so that many of us live on 'low-fat' diets consistently, believing that fats add nothing but calories to our food. With this 'fat phobia' on the upsweep it is imperative to recognize the difference between *good fats* and *bad fats*.

Traditionally, oils were mechanically cold-pressed in small amounts for immediate consumption, and distributed to local households in much the same way as the milkman brings fresh milk. The reason for this was that fats turn rancid quickly. We now have refrigeration and chemical methods that prolong the shelf life of these oils. However, the fats we consume today are fundamentally different from those consumed in the not-so-distant past. Industrialization has brought about large-scale production of oils, and now huge expeller oil-presses have replaced the smaller, slower, cold-temperature mechanical presses of the past. Modern technologies have found new methods of processing that allow manufacturers to produce cheap, low-quality oils with a longer shelf life.

So what happens when we heat oils? When we *heat* fats we upset their delicate balance. **The heating process alters the molecular structures of fats, producing free radicals (destructive molecular fragments that are formed during metabolism).** Heating at high temperatures turns these oils into twisted molecules called trans-fatty acids. The heat causes the fatty acid bonds to break down, creating free radicals in the form of short-chain fatty acids, trans-fats, and saturated fats. These fats are all too happy to react with oxygen, and when rapid oxidation occurs it increases the dangers to our health. These unnatural fats are toxic and can interfere with cell function and the use of oxygen in the body. Exposing *good fats* to heat will destroy their long carbon-chain bonds and change them to short-chain fatty acids, thus changing them to trans- and saturated fats. These heated unnatural fats leave us wide open to the increased danger of free-radical damage – which may cause an array of pathogenic problems. Oils prepared in this damaging way are better known as hydrogenated or partially hydrogenated oils. These types of oil now become more shelf stable at room temperature, which for commercial reasons is far more profitable. You will find hydrogenated oils and partially hydrogenated oils in bakery products, frozen foods, margarines and many more products on the market – so check your labels.

Is there such a thing as 'safe frying'? Well, there is consistent evidence that shows fried fats cause hardening of the arteries and makes blood platelets sticky. Frying, deep-fat frying and sautéing are the most popular methods of using oils and fats today. Deep-fried fast food is cooked in oils that have often been used repeatedly. The foods are then submerged in these dangerous oils. Subjecting foods to this destructive practice is definitely *not* good for your health. Because heated oils are so damaging to our health you will find *none* of these oils in my recipes. That's right, not even olive oil, except the cold-pressed, unrefined and unheated kind. Virgin olive oil has many benefits and healing powers. It protects the cardiovascular system and has anti-mutagenic properties, but it too is susceptible to heat and oxidation damage and the benefits come only from oil that is cold-pressed, unrefined and unheated. Keep this in mind the next time you prepare a meal.

Instead of using heated oils, I have chosen small amounts of butter or coconut fat for some of the recipes because of their stability at high temperatures. Frying or sautéing is not a practice I recommend; try to use water to sauté your food and add the fats after the food is removed from the heat source. **I use Udo's oil for various recipes in salad dressings, smoothies and patés because it is a rich source of omega 3, 6 and 9.** Because this oil is made from seeds its taste does not overpower the food.

By this stage you should be starting to get the picture that the wheels of commercialism and large-scale profits are of far more interest to producers than our nutritional needs. As our health is based on the amount of absorbable nutrition we provide our bodies, it is necessary to get back to some grass-root solutions if we are to solve the problems left in the wake of our impoverished diets.

I rest my case now, so let's get on with the enjoyable pleasure of making some delicious food!

Nature's Pharmacy

It can be difficult to figure out which supplements are the most effective and the best value for money. When we live on a mediocre diet, we need to supplement with effective and absorbable nutrients.

Powerful Supplements

There are so many supplements on the market these days that it can be difficult to figure out which ones are most effective, and which are the best value for money. I have found the scientific evidence to be a minefield of contradictions, and I believe firmly that it is of more benefit to get high doses of nutrients direct from Mother Nature through juicing and eating the proper foods. While it might be tempting to believe that popping some vitamin pills is the easiest way to compensate for a poor or mediocre diet, this is not the case. **Nutrients must be supplied in a way that the body can readily assimilate otherwise they will be of little benefit.** I am often asked my opinion on supplements. The following are some of the supplements that I use and have found effective and, most important of all, absorbable.

Enzymes

I have already mentioned enzymes in so many sections of this book that I'm sure by now you have a picture of how important they are to our overall health. **Digestive enzymes are like a knife that chops the foods we eat into smaller, more usable nutrients that support the cells, tissues, organs and glands of the entire body.**

Although a high proportion of the foods I eat are uncooked, I still use enzyme supplements every day. Enzyme supplementation is extremely important for those eating a regular diet of cooked foods. When we eat live/enzyme-rich foods in the form of juices, sprouts and raw food, this saves the body from using up its own precious enzymes and frees up the body to concentrate on the important task of protecting the immune system. In fact, many experts believe that the health of an individual can be evaluated by analysing their enzyme status.

Enzymes are powerful for providing healing processes within the body. They contribute to every chemical and muscle action in the body, from digestion to the repair of damaged tissue. If we do not supply adequate amounts of enzymes to the body, all too often the result is food allergies, wind, bloating, digestive upsets, weakened immunity and low energy levels. Enzymes play a major role in all the body's systems and protect our cells from free-radical damage. These molecular fragments (free radicals) not only damage health but are also instrumental in accelerating the process of ageing. Enzymes slow down the ageing process, although keep in mind that while they protect our bodies from the ageing process they will not reverse it (wishful thinking!). Many of the people I know who use enzymes tell me they would use them for that reason alone.

There are two main sources of enzymes: internal and external.

Internally the digestive system secretes enzymes in saliva, gastric juices and in the pancreas and intestine. External enzymes are best found in raw foods. Nature endows all raw food with the enzymes required for digestion. As you have seen in previous chapters, modern food-processing techniques and cooking methods destroy almost 100 per cent of the enzymes needed for the vital job of breaking down and absorbing food. You have also seen that today's Western diet no longer contains as much raw food as the diet of previous generations. The combination of cooked food, alcohol, stress and micronutrient deficiencies all take their toll on the body's enzymes reserves. This is especially noticeable as we age and begin to produce fewer digestive enzymes.

Enzyme insufficiency puts enormous strain on our digestive system, and this in turn causes acid reflux, indigestion and constipation. People battling serious digestive problems can obtain excellent results in a relatively short time when they supplement their diet with good-quality digestive enzymes. Throughout the initial stages of chemotherapy I found it very difficult to keep down and digest food. I then learned about the important role of digestive enzymes and I began to supplement my diet. The results were immediate and I began to eat normally within three days of starting to take these supplements.

When purchasing enzyme supplements make sure you choose a 100 per cent plant-based enzyme. Plant-based enzymes have a wide range of activity throughout the entire digestive tract and assist in aiding and completing the digestive process. Look for a product that contains protein-digesting enzymes (protease). These formulas work in the acidic pH of the stomach and will deliver the most complete digestion. Protease-rich formulas are also effective at helping the body deal with colds and infections, and they can be taken on an empty stomach to help boost the immune system. Use as many enzymes as necessary to optimize digestion, and remember that everyone can benefit from using digestive enzymes to improve digestion and nutrient absorption. As enzymes have no taste the capsules can simply be opened and sprinkled on cold or warm (but not hot) food. This powerful and effective supplement is at the very top of my list.

Essential Fats

Many people consider Omega 3, Omega 6 and Omega 9 fats as supplements. This, of course, is not true as their source is mainly from foods. Omega fats are major nutrients that should be used in tablespoon amounts, and not in milligrams. **We need more of these essential fatty acids every day than we do of any other nutrient.** Essential fats are so important because they are required for the healthy functioning of every cell, tissue, gland and organ in our bodies.

I am often told of the difficulties people experience when trying to increase their intake of these *vital* essential fats. Well, I'm not surprised some people find it difficult to swallow large amounts of oil straight from a spoon! Integrating these good fats into foods is much easier and makes the fats more absorbable. As fats improve the flavour of food, they should be introduced into the diet wherever possible. I use these good fats in sandwiches, dressings, or drizzled over potatoes or vegetables. Please remember that your body cannot make these essential fats by itself, so it is absolutely necessary that you provide the body with good amounts of these essential nutrients in the foods you eat.

Probiotics

Probiotics are the beneficial bacteria that naturally occur along the intestinal tract. They are absolutely essential for a proper digestive system, strong immune function, and good overall health. Friendly bacteria constantly compete with unfriendly micro-organisms that enter our system, and can multiply within the body, causing many problems. When the ratio of good bacteria is lowered, it increases the risk of yeast overgrowths and fungal infections. **The use of antibiotics in the production of non-organic meats, dairy products and farmed fish, as well as pharmaceutical medical treatments, can wreak havoc on the delicate balance of our gastrointestinal tract and immune system.** Once destroyed, these beneficial bacteria can only be replaced through supplementation because the body cannot regenerate them on its own.

Of course you can obtain friendly bacteria from yoghurt, but most yoghurt will only provide millions of one particular strain of bacteria. These products are not good value for money if you are looking to provide large amounts of good bacteria to the entire body. The reason for this is because the digestive tract requires many different strains of these friendly bacteria. To provide the mouth, gums, oesophagus, stomach, small intestine and large intestine with sufficient good bacteria it is necessary to use a good probiotic supplement that will effectively establish large healthy populations of friendly bacteria. **Optimum colonization can be easily achieved with a high-strength probiotic supplement which contains a wide range of lactobacteria for the upper intestines and a bifidobacteria for the lower intestines.**

Probiotics enhance the immune system's ability to prevent unfriendly organisms, such as salmonella and *E. coli*, from gaining a foothold within the body. These effective supplements can also be of great benefit for a wide variety of conditions, such as colitis and Irritable Bowel Syndrome. They can be taken orally or can also be used externally to combat a variety of yeast and fungal infections. For example; the capsules can be broken open and the contents placed in socks for protection against athlete's foot. Likewise, vaginal micro-flora can improve with the supplementation of probiotics, and infections such as thrush and *Candida albicans* can be treated quickly and successfully. Again, the contents of the capsules need simply be placed in underwear and taken orally to relieve the symptoms of these infections.

Probiotics work best when placed in the mouth, and offer effective protection against tooth decay and help to keep bad breath at bay. These supplements can impair the growth and activity of the harmful ulcer-causing *H. pylori* bacteria and will also protect against the harmful effects of radiation and pollutants. **Probiotics should be taken daily to ensure replacement of the bacteria killed by poor eating habits.** They should be taken in increased amounts before, during and after prescribed antibiotics. When travelling you should take probiotics with you for protection against problematic micro-organisms that may be found in food and water.

Keep your probiotics refrigerated whenever possible. This is an important fact to remember when storing and buying probiotics, as refrigeration ensures maximum potency and stability. They should only be left unrefrigerated for short periods of time. Probiotics work best if taken immediately after meals, when the acidity of the gastric juices has been diluted by food. Lactic bacteria are sensitive to extreme acidity and therefore their passage through the stomach is easier when gastric juices are not as concentrated. I use probiotics regularly for myself and my family, and consider them an absolute must.

Blue-green Algae

Blue-green algae are powerful natural multi-nutrient supplements. They are often referred to as green superfoods. Synthetic manufactured multivitamin and -mineral supplements often come in a form that the body cannot absorb easily. Algae grow naturally and have a well-balanced range of many essential vitamins and minerals, amino acids and live enzymes in an organic form that is readily absorbed by the human body. Blue-green algae share characteristics with plants, animals and bacteria, and this is what makes them so highly absorbable for humans. Since these algae grow naturally, the human body recognizes them as food that is easily absorbed through the intestinal walls. This makes all their vital nutrients totally accessible for absorption by the body – just as nature intended.

Blue-green algae are some of the Earth's finest living organisms. For thousands of years they have been an important food source for human populations. The ancient Aztecs harvested them from the Mexican mountain lakes to use for trading purposes. They mixed the algae with maize to provide a nutritious meal. Today the Kanembus tribe in Chad, Africa still regularly uses algae.

Unlike other tribes in the region, the children of this tribe show no signs of malnutrition.

Many of us suffer from poor nutrient absorption caused by a sluggish body, a liver overloaded by toxins and a malfunctioning digestive system. Nutrient-deficient processed foods only add to the problem. These problems deplete the body's store of nutrients, and this is why a good absorbable supplement is necessary. Some of the best algae available are found in the upper Kalmath Lake in Oregon, USA, where the mineral deposits from volcanic lava flow into this 140-square-mile lake. The natural ideal conditions of this unique lake provide a rich source of nutrients of superior quality. Kalmath blue-green algae is certified organic. **Many scientists consider blue-green algae to be the most nutrient-rich food source on the planet.** This truly is an excellent absorbable nutrient.

Grape Seed Extract

Grape seed has been identified as a potent antioxidant that protects our cells from free radical damage. Dr Jacques Masquelier, a research scientist at the University of Bordeaux in France, made a significant discovery in nutritional science by isolating a powerful antioxidant known as OPGs (Oligomeric Proantho Cyanidins) which neutralizes free-radical molecules. These destructive scavengers have been identified to contribute to cell destruction, and because cell damage is the root cause of most health problems and eating disorders, protecting ourselves from free-radical activity is a significant preventative measure for a long and healthy life. **Grape seed extract is more powerful than vitamin C in its ability to scavenge free radicals.**

Beyond this, grape seed also helps to strengthen the entire vascular system and helps prevent capillary leakage in the legs, eyes and skin. It also is effective at reducing fluid retention. Free radicals degenerate these vessels, causing lesions that become traps for bad cholesterol (LDL). Once (LDL) cholesterol has been trapped in this manner, it attracts calcium. Cholesterol and calcium build up to form a plaque which narrows the arteries and encourages blood-clot formation. Grape seed extract provides nutritional support for a healthy heart and so can help to maintain normal blood flow.

Grape seed extract also strengthens collagen fibres (a tough flexible protein). Collagen is an essential and major component of muscles, ligaments, teeth, gums, eyes and blood vessels. Collagen is the protein constituent of connective tissue that exists throughout the body in pairs of strands. Hydrogen bridges connect these strands and give collagen its strength. **The protective action of grape seed extract strengthens collagen protein, which improves elasticity and resiliency.** As we age we lose the elasticity in the skin because we have fewer collagen fibres. Collagen that is weak and inflexible contributes to premature ageing. Grape seed extract can help reduce the visible signs of premature ageing, such as wrinkles and sagging skin. It helps avert premature ageing by reducing free-radical-induced weakening of collagen. This powerful antioxidant supports the body's ability to maintain and enhance the health of connective tissue, and the elasticity of the skin. Although this substance cannot completely prevent the ageing process, it is probably more effective than many of the costly anti-ageing creams available on the market. It is also useful in helping eliminate age spots caused by sun damage. Absorption of this powerful antioxidant begins 10 minutes after entering the digestive tract, and maximum absorption is reached within 45 minutes. This powerful antioxidant delivers significant health benefits and skin benefits which makes including it in our diet well worthwhile.

Step Three: Water – Pure and Simple

Water is a necessity for life, but it is also necessary to ensure the water we drink is clean …

Water Should Just Be Water

You may well be appalled when you discover the chemical cocktail that the average water supply actually contains. Preventing tooth decay by adding fluoride to our water makes very little sense when it creates an unacceptable toxic health hazard.

One of the biggest concerns for health is that of the quality of the water we drink. Nowadays we spend time and money carrying bottled water into our homes because we fear contamination of our tap water supply. But why go to this bother when we can easily clean the water coming into our homes? You may well be appalled when you discover the chemical cocktail that the average water supply actually contains. One thing is for sure – it does not make for happy reading! But just as water is a necessity for life, it is also necessary to ensure the water we drink is clean. Let's have a look at our need for water, the problems with water, and also how we can clean the water that comes into our homes.

The Body's Need for Water

We now have a much greater awareness that a sufficient quantity of clean water is absolutely necessary to keep us healthy. The importance of drinking clean water regularly cannot be stressed highly enough. Water is the crucial agent which flushes out toxins, aids digestion and also prevents premature ageing and disease in the cells of our bodies. The lymph system requires clean water to assist in its daily functions of eliminating waste and debris from the body.

It is actually relatively easy to become dehydrated, especially when you are regularly drinking coffee, tea or sugary fizzy drinks. Drinking these beverages does the exact opposite of hydrating the body. They will cause the body to lose water and can even be responsible for leaching essential nutrients from the body. The process of adjusting your body to drinking larger amounts of water is a gradual process, and can be made easier by adding some lemon juice and warming it to body temperature; this will help you to consume those extra few glasses. As water cleanses your system internally, it is vital for healthy glowing skin. Insufficient hydration of the body can lead to a breakdown in the cell structure of the skin, which results in premature ageing and sagging skin. Another upside to drinking water consistently is that it increases your metabolism and will also help to control your weight.

A huge variety of illnesses – including asthma and ulcers, high blood pressure and arthritis, a general feeling of lethargy, headaches, tiredness and constipation – are all contributed to by a lack of a regular and sufficient supply of clean water to the body. Hydrating the body with fresh juices and clean water is also an essential tool for fighting cancer.

The Problems with Water

Bottled Water

Do you feel that bottled water is a rip off? Apart from the inflated prices and expense of bottled water, there are a few facts you should familiarize yourself with before you part with your cash.

We mistakenly believe that drinking bottled mineral water will meet the body's requirements for vital minerals. The simple fact is that water *neither takes nor gives nutrition,* as the body's need for minerals is met through plant foods. Plants pick up mineral elements from the soil and make these minerals available to us through the foods we eat. Minerals in this form are compatible with the needs of our cells, and it is *only* minerals which are compatible with the cells that will be utilized by the body. Unless the body can utilize the minerals in the water, the body's cells will reject them. This can leave accumulations of excess minerals in the body that can clog up the cells and organs. These deposits can accumulate in arteries, veins, joints and muscles.

Another problem we are now exposed to lies in the plastic bottles that hold the water. A student of mine was advised by her doctors to take her seven-year-old daughter off bottled mineral water after she developed kidney stones. This is typical of the obstructions that these calcifications cause. Soft plastic bottles are also toxic and can leach oestrogens and other substances into the water.

Tap Water

Have you ever wondered what exactly is in our water supply? **Just because the water coming out of your tap looks clear and transparent, this does not mean that it is actually clean.**

Like mineral water, tap water also contains hard deposits. These deposits pass from the intestinal walls into the lymphatic system and to all parts of the body, which can cause hardening of the arteries, calcification of the blood vessels and kidney stones. In much the same way as your kettle builds up stone-like calcifications of lime, these deposits gather within the filtering apparatus of the kidneys, because every drop of water that comes into the body must pass through this system.

It is inexcusable that we are given no choice as to the chemical treatment procedures that expose us to hazardous chemicals such as fluoride in our water supply. This toxic chemical certainly does not warrant a place in our drinking water. Let's have a brief look at some of the major toxic contaminants.

Chlorine

Chlorine is a gas that is added to the water supply in order to kill germs. It is used for fumigating, bleaching and disinfecting. This cheap disinfectant is used primarily to kill harmful bacteria. While it is of course necessary for water-treatment plants to kill off germs, viruses and bacteria, unfortunately there are major drawbacks with these procedures. These chemicals do not

destroy microbes such as *E. coli* and *Cryptosporidium*, as many of
these strains have become resistant to them. What's more is that
chlorine is also responsible for destroying good bacteria as well
as harmful bacteria. Only a fraction of the microscopically-spread
waterborne illnesses are reported, and incidences of infections
from these organisms have soared. Interference from chlorination
and fluoridation of water can also denature enzymes. As already
outlined, enzymes are crucial in assisting all functions of the
body and are the essence of life. My little daughter Julie
remarked to me how tap water smells like a swimming pool.
How true this is. The unpleasant taste and smell are among the
reasons why so many people are reluctant to drink it and end up
being dehydrated.

Fluoride

There is no scientific evidence to prove any of the proposed
benefits of fluoride. Fluoride is a substance which has never been
approved for human consumption in any country in the world.
The chief chemist from the US National Cancer Institute – Dr
Dean Burk – has conducted large epidemiological studies into
fluoridated water and states that fluoride causes more human
cancer deaths than any other chemical. This toxic substance is
only slightly less toxic than arsenic and has never been safety-
tested on humans. To date it has been rejected and banned by 23
EU member states.

The issue of adding this poisonous insecticide, which is
commonly used in rat poison formulations, to our drinking water

97

has caused uproar over the past few decades. Even dentists took a dim view of its use before it was introduced. Yet fluoride is still used extensively! When this issue raises its ugly head by those opposing fluoridation, the subject is quickly defused. If the United States FDA (Food and Drug Administration) have seen it fit to accentuate its toxicity by placing a warning on toothpaste labels, surely this substance should no longer be entering our drinking water. Fluoride is a by-product of aluminium and contains high concentrations of heavy metals such as lead, arsenic and chromium – all proven carcinogens (cancer-causing agents). Exposure to such carcinogens can bring about metabolic and biochemical changes to all living tissue. Long-term ingestion of fluoride can accumulate in the skeleton, joints and glands, and is also linked to Irritable Bowel Syndrome, cancer, arthritis and osteoporosis.

Preventing tooth decay by adding fluoride to our water makes very little sense as it creates an unacceptable toxic health hazard. Are we to believe our overall health is irrelevant as long as our teeth are free of cavities? **A recent report for the UK Department of Health and Social Security stated that 'no essential function exists for fluoride in the diet.'** The truth is that bacteria is what causes cavities, not a lack of fluoride, and good dental hygiene is the safer answer.

On top of these two listed chemicals there are many other harmful substances such as aluminium, arsenic, cadmium, lead and nitrates in our water that would take up more time to explain than we have available in this book. You will see from this brief synopsis that the water we drink is undeniably unsafe for human consumption. It follows, then, that we need to consider carefully all the available data and establish better methods of cleaning our water. We also need to curtail the widespread exposure to these dangerous chemicals. For me, when diagnosed with cancer I had no time to waste for governments or water authorities to clean up their act, so I had to set about cleaning the water coming into my home. The following two systems are effective ways of doing just this.

How Clean Is Your Water?

Jug filters are not very effective at filtering chemicals and microbes from water. In fact they are a breeding ground for bacteria. These filters merely use a screen to separate only particles of dirt sediment from water. The two most effective systems for this filtering process are steamed distillation or filtration through a reverse-osmosis system.

Distilled Water

Some people believe that distilled water leaches minerals from the body. This assumption is inaccurate because in fact distilled water acts like a sponge that removes minerals which cannot be utilized by the body. Using a home distiller will give you clean water free of contaminants. Tap water is heated to 100°C, a temperature at which bacteria, germs, viruses and cysts can be killed. The steam rises, leaving behind dissolved solids, chemicals, salts, contaminants and impurities. This steam then condenses into distilled water – which is water just about as clean as you can get it. These distillers are readily available in portable, compact units (at the lower price range), or larger more permanent units (which are higher priced).

Reverse Osmosis

This filtration system is cost effective and uses the principle of reverse osmosis to remove 95–98 per cent of all the mineral and chemical contaminants from raw tap water. Reverse osmosis was originally designed to make seawater drinkable for the Navy. As you can imagine, it would be imperative for the Navy to have its own mobile purification system to eliminate storage of vast amounts of water. This filtration system operates when a membrane separates a salt-water solution and a water solution. The water will pass through the membrane to reach the salt, in order to achieve equilibrium. This is the process by which our cells absorb nutrients. In one of these systems, by reversing the process, the two are separated again – salt and contaminants on one side, pure water on the other. Reverse osmosis uses a semi-permeable membrane that removes not only particles but an extremely high percentage of dissolved contaminant molecules from water. In this first-class processing system, five separate filters remove dirt, rust, chlorine, chemicals, multi-chemical compounds, micro-organisms and bacteria. The system fits under the sink unit and has a separate tap that is easily installed on your kitchen counter or sink, and gives you an unlimited supply of good drinking water. This system is easy to maintain, and the filters need to be changed only once a year. It should be noted also that filtering systems with one or two filters will not filter out microbes, as these microbes are too small for these inferior systems.

Both these systems will give you water which is clean, fresh, tastes good and is more economical and convenient than buying bottled water. Thanks to the purity of the water produced by these systems they are used for kidney dialysis and within medical and pharmaceutical laboratories – which stands as a good indication of how effective both these systems are. Check the Resources section at the end of this book for a source to find a system to suit you.

Step Four: What's Not on the Label?

*Should we go with the flow or wake up
and smell the chemicals?*

Safe Personal Care

Take the time to get informed, purchase wisely and use products that will keep you safe, because after all ... You know you're worth it.

Many of us are completely unaware of the potentially harmful chemicals used in everyday products like toothpaste, shampoo, deodorant, moisturizers, body lotions and makeup. We buy these products in good faith and assume they are safe to use, but unfortunately this is not the case. How trusting we are with the numerous products we massage into our skin, spray onto our armpits, scrub our teeth and gums with, and clean our babies with. Yet the long-term effects of many of these chemicals are unknown. Because we are the first generation to be exposed to the dangers of using these harmful substances, only time will tell what the consequences and the adverse effects on the population will be. It's up to the consumer to take the time to consider these issues and weigh up the pros and cons, and decide if the means justify the end.

We don't give a moment's thought to the impact exposure to cancer-causing ingredients in these everyday, familiar products has on our health. On the other hand, the cosmetic industry spends both time and money (billions of dollars to be precise) persuading us that we *need* their products. Their sophisticated advertising techniques not only persuade us to buy their products, but also try to convince us that many of their products are a basic necessity. Look at how these advertisements prey on our fears that we are not taking proper care of our bodies, and often in a way that makes us feel very vulnerable.

We may well believe that our bodies will betray us at the wrong moment with unwanted bad smells. Quite frankly, this type of advertising does a very good job of putting enough effective pressure on us to make us part with our hard-earned cash. So what are we to do? Are we, the consuming public, prepared to sit by passively and allow this industry to get away with bombarding us with hazardous chemicals? **Should we go with the flow or wake up and smell the chemicals?** These major multinational companies may well argue it is not their intent to corrupt their products with harmful ingredients. Once they list the ingredients they fulfil their role; it is entirely up to us consumers to decide if we want to purchase these products. Once again, the choice is ours.

You Know It Makes Sense – Common Sense

Scrutinizing and checking labels is not an easy process for those of us who are not in the know. It's of little benefit being confronted with a list of complicated ingredients that is difficult to understand. It can be difficult to get to grips with incomprehensible labels typed in the smallest possible print, and we automatically switch off to the information displayed right in front of us. When it comes to anti-ageing creams, most of us are dubious enough despite the slick miraculous marketing claims. Clever marketing also takes advantage by trying to reassure us with meaningless terms such as 'natural', 'organic' and 'hypo-allergenic'. It may at first seem reassuring to see these labels, but this untrustworthy language is misleading and often masks the truth behind these prettily packaged toiletries and cosmetics. Unfortunately most of us believe that these terms could not be used if they were not true, when in fact, for example, 'hypo-allergenic' simply means the manufacturer feels it is *less likely* to cause allergic reactions.

Here again there are ongoing opportunities to make large profits, as these products often command a high price. We believe that they have unique specific natural formulations that are of a superior quality to 'normal' products. **We have to remind ourselves again that where there are vested interests, responsibility for the consumer's long-term health is not always on the agenda.** There is no doubt that there are many questions to be answered about the safety of the ingredients in these everyday personal care products. The next few paragraphs will give you a starting point and may well convince you that you need to make informed choices when it comes to your personal care products.

Let's first have a look at some key information on the dangerous chemicals that exist in everyday personal care products. (In the

Resources section you'll find suppliers for user-healthy alternatives to these products.)

Toothpaste

Most of us would gasp at the thought that a product as familiar as toothpaste can contain harmful ingredients such as fluoride and sodium lauryl sulphate. If you take the time to check the precise ingredients on the average tube of toothpaste, you may well decide you need to change your choice of products. We are well aware that children often swallow toothpaste because of its sweet taste. This sweetness is the result of the use of artificial sweeteners such as saccharin, a known carcinogen (a cancer-causing substance).

As most people recognize the fact that toothpaste contains fluoride, I think I should bring your attention to a few more facts about this chemical. If as little as 1 gram of fluoride is ingested, it can cause dangerous poisoning. Fluoride can accumulate in body tissue and can be poisonous if ingested over long periods of time (WHO Geneva: World Health Organization Fluoride and Dental Health 1994).

By law, all toothpaste sold in America must carry a warning sign which states clearly 'If more than what is needed for brushing is accidentally swallowed, contact a poisons control centre immediately.'

This is toothpaste we are talking about! This is that familiar product that we use twice daily in our mouths. US labelling laws are 15 years ahead of the labelling laws that exist here in the UK and Ireland, and are much more stringent. Upon investigation I discovered that safety data sheets actually list sodium fluoride as a *severe poison*. When you consider the risks from this substance, surely it would be wiser to find a safer alternative.

Shampoo

The main offenders in commercial shampoos are the harsh synthetic detergents that are listed as sodium lauryl sulphate or sodium laureth sulphate. These irritating foaming agents are also found in toothpaste and children's bubble bath. Sodium lauryl sulphate is an aggressive cleaner that is the most reported common cause of eye irritations in commercial shampoos. It has a low molecular weight that is rapidly absorbed by the body and will readily penetrate the skin. When ingested it is more toxic than if it were taken intravenously. It is also retained in the eyes, brain and liver – particularly in the eyes of the young – and its effect on the liver and brain are cumulative. Skin allergies, contact eczema and cataracts (and also mouth ulcers in the case of toothpaste) are some of the risks we are exposing ourselves to when we use this harsh chemical.

Sodium *laureth* sulphate is widely used in most children's shampoos, as it is somewhat milder. Sodium laureth sulphate can contain 1-4 dioxane (a potent toxin), which is a known carcinogen. If you have concerns about these harmful chemicals in your shampoo and toothpaste, you may want to reduce your exposure to their harmful effects by becoming a more selective shopper.

Antiperspirants/Deodorants

The main culprit found in antiperspirant deodorants is aluminium. Aluminium compounds are neurotoxic for humans and have a build-up effect in the brain, liver and lungs. This is very evident when we look at the research into Alzheimer's disease, which found that large amounts of aluminium were contained in the brains of sufferers. The link with Alzheimer's disease and aluminium compounds has been scientifically proven. When we use products that contain these harmful substances, the liver must work harder to try to rid the body of them. These detrimental foreign substances can become entwined in DNA and can cause damage at a cellular level. Products containing aluminium compounds are listed as known or suspected carcinogens (Cornell Carcinogens Database). It should also be noted that cancer and osteoporosis are other dangers associated with these chemical cocktails.

The US FDA advisory panel has called for the removal of these chemicals from antiperspirant deodorants. Many harmful substances that were considered safe to use in the past had catastrophic side-effects for humans and are now banned. So bear in mind that the invisible dangers contained in the products we are now exposing ourselves to may well become the banned substances of tomorrow. When it comes to antiperspirants, my belief is that less is always best.

Skincare Products

Many of us believe that our skin forms an effective barrier that will protect the body against harmful substances. However, if we look into the matter it is easy to see that the skin is not an effective barrier. This is evident when we look at products such as nicotine patches that are used to ease withdrawal symptoms associated with nicotine addiction. These trans-dermal delivery systems utilize the skin's unique ability to transport molecules into the bloodstream. **In exactly the same way, harmful chemicals found in the skincare products can be absorbed and diffused across membranes, and can enter into the bloodstream.**

Propylene glycol is a substance found in many skincare products, makeup, body lotion, baby wipes and hair products. This substance is a strong skin irritant that many people have sensitivities towards; it may be a potential culprit if you are suffering from itchy or irritated skin. Propylene glycol prevents the evaporation of moisture, thus giving the skin a younger appearance. When we use this in skincare preparations, the outer layers of skin cells absorb more water; this in turn makes the skin cells swell similar to the way a dried prune placed in water begins to swell.

This form of hydration may sound quite appealing at first, but you may not relish the thought quite so much when you consider that this substance is also found in paint, liquid laundry detergents, antifreeze and brake fluid. Listed as a suspected neurotoxicity hazard by the EDF (Environmental Defence Fund), propylene glycol can weaken the immune system and has been found to cause kidney damage and liver abnormalities. Safety data sheets supplied with this product when this chemical is used for industrial use stipulate that the user must *avoid* contact with the skin. If you are encountering skin irritations you should try to break your dependence on the products that contain propylene glycol and adopt a new skincare regime.

Much of the information I have presented to you is underreported in the media. **The World Wildlife Foundation are fighting to get the chemical industry regulated better so that the worst of these chemicals are phased out or replaced with safer alternatives.** The WWF tested the blood of some well-known celebrities and found without exception that their blood was laden with toxic chemicals. A synopsis of these results is available at www.wwf.org.uk. What is obvious is that we need to open our eyes to this information and educate ourselves on the dangers that these potentially harmful chemicals pose to our health. We also need to make some wise decisions when purchasing personal care products. Although this may paint a bleak picture of the products you might currently use, there are many safe alternatives available from health stores, on-line, or from distributors (see the Resources chapter). Rest assured that it is relatively simple to switch to safe personal care toiletries.

Remember, when it comes to personal care products you can change your mind at any time and simply buy your products elsewhere. Above all else, you should take the time to become informed, purchase wisely, and use products that will keep you safe because, after all …

You know you're worth it.

A Final Note …

Nutritious food serves as an investment in the future and the best health insurance policy you can get your hands on.

I hope this book has provided you with the motivation and inspiration to make changes for the better to your diet. Believe me, your body will thank you for it. If you decide to step up to the mark and make the choice to be kinder to your body, it will be important not to be swayed by excuses or criticism from others. The voice of disapproval from others will inevitably come before, during and after you make your decision. The phrase 'you only live once' is just one of the many excuses you will have to become accustomed to as you try to improve your diet. Remember, that's exactly what you are trying to do – live once. You may well be labelled as fussy or different because you don't eat 'normal' foods. But if the truth be told, some of those critics may actually envy your ability to make changes that they themselves would find difficult even to contemplate. Be prepared to anticipate negative responses and be conscious that we all have human frailties – but stick to your own beliefs. **Your body will intuitively show you what foods are best for you, and will be very grateful for the fundamental and practical steps you are taking to maximize your potential for optimum health.** In time you may well be awarded grudging respect for your decision, and you might eventually encourage others to phase some positive changes into their own lives.

The golden rule is consistency. This is an absolute must if you are to succeed in transforming unhealthy and addictive eating habits and improve the quality of both your health and your life.

Lifestyle changes can be quite empowering, and sometimes it can be difficult to curb your enthusiasm – especially when eating with family and friends. Attempting to persuade your nearest and dearest to 'clean up their act' can be hard work. So remember that sometimes, no matter how well intentioned you are, they may feel you are judging or criticizing their eating choices. Believe me, initially I made many mistakes in this area and I well remember the arguments that raged around my kitchen table. Bear in mind that it is difficult to change the eating habits of a lifetime, particularly if not motivated by some particular reason.

Eating with family and friends is an immensely pleasurable and bonding experience, so changing their eating habits can sometimes require tolerance and a lot of negotiation. Changing their diet for the better is not something that is going to happen overnight. So be aware that those who come on board straight away tend to be in the minority. Do your best to enlist their support, as this will encourage them to eat more healthily and will help to avoid conflict. Conflict is the last thing you want during this transition period. You can't expect others to jump in feet first along with you, but by leading from the front your example may eventually influence them. From my own experience, appealing to their taste buds is the only way to go.

We all enjoy eating good food; however, the biggest failing of the people of today's developed world is that we turn this pleasure into junk/binge eating that can only serve to make us sick in the future. It seems ludicrous to me that we continue to overfeed ourselves and ignore the impact of our distinctly unhealthy Western diet on our health. Why do we continue to subject ourselves to the misery of the increasing epidemic of food-related diseases? Heart disease, cancer, diabetes, irritable bowel syndrome, arthritis … the list is endless.

Changing our eating habits may well be the biggest and most important challenge facing us, but one thing is for sure – long-term change is an absolute must. **Nutritious food serves as an investment in the future and the best health insurance policy you can get your hands on.** If changing your eating patterns brings about positive and obvious good effects on your body, then I say 'Go for it'. This way at least you are back in the driving seat.

I hope this programme will encourage you to become more informed and more familiar with the basic facts about food and our bodies. We certainly have a great deal to learn about the important role of food, and the preparation of food, in the creation of good health. By discovering a few key truths we can make a huge difference to our mostly ignored state of health.

When we are not trying to help or cure a specific condition, we rarely prioritize and take the time to invest in the lifestyle changes necessary for good health. We all too often become guilty of the 'I'll start on Monday' syndrome. The time is NOW and I cannot stress enough to you that *prevention is always better than cure*. Waiting for an illness to be your incentive can sometimes be too little too late.

The recipes that follow are neither virtuous nor self-indulgent. They are just honest-to-goodness real food from nature's kitchen – food that is available to all of us. It is not written in stone that we have to stick with well-known addictive foods. It is not fixed that we cannot open our minds to new ideas and provide our bodies with good solid nourishment which will lead to better health. We can then give in to our desire for an occasional treat without guilt. Remember that with these vital building blocks for survival and growth come endless opportunities for true health. Mother Nature will pay you back in earnest if you follow her guidelines and bring your diet back to its grass-roots.

It is truly possible.

Be well.

The Recipes

I hope you will enjoy the easy preparation and delicious taste that will contribute to a more vibrant, healthier you …

Juices

Smoothies

Breakfasts

No-cook Soups

Super Rich Broccoli and Almond Soup   155

Asian Seaweed Soup   156

Fresh Tomato and Basil Soup   157

Cooked Soups

Heart-warming Protein-rich Soup   161

Butternut Squash, Coconut and Chilli Bean Soup   162

Sweet Potato and Lemongrass Soup   164

Fresh Main Meals

Vegetable Stir Raw with Ginger and Almond Dressing   169

Unfried Italian-style Vegetables   170

Red Pepper Ragu Sauce   171

Tasty Pizza Base   172

Health Nut's Cream Cheese   174

Savoury Sweetcorn Pancakes   175

East Meets West Falafel   176

Fresh Crunchy Kebabs   177

Cooked Main Meals

Pinto Bean Sweet Potato Stew with Lemon Mint Pesto   180

Leek Pie with Roast Garlic and Butter Bean Mash   182

Vegetable Ragout with Herb Spaghetti   184

Sweet Potato and Broccoli Sambar   186

Puy Lentil and Spinach Stew   188

Tuscan-style Peppers   190

Snacks

Fabulous Lunch Patties   195

Energy Wraps with Garlic Dill Sauce   196

Corn on the Cob with Sassy Salsa   197

Gosia's Powerful Paté   198

Omega-rich Sprouted Sandwich   199

Zucchini Sandwiches   200

Mediterranean Flax Crackers   201

Sun-kissed Basil Pesto   202

Ripe Guacamole Dip   203

Spicy Curry Crackers   204

Get Stuffed Tomatoes   205

Hearty Stuffed Mushrooms   206

Sides

No-grain Tabbouleh   209

Thai Parsnip Rice   210

Golden Couscous   211

Salads

Mixed Herb Salad with Spicy Sunflower Seeds   215

Crisp Baby Spinach Leaves with Garlic Mushrooms   216

Slurpy Tomato and Onion Salad   217

Marinated Broccoli with Sprouted Sesame Seeds   218

No-cook Tasty Treats

Baked Treats

Juices

*Juices are highly concentrated
forms of nutrition …*

Irresistible Grape

serves 1

The incredibly sweet taste of this juice is a must if you are new to juicing. I always introduce this juice first in my classes because of its enticing taste. It is a wonderful way to increase your fruit intake. Grapes contain selenium, zinc and are a good source of antioxidants, which help to fight the ageing process. Be sure to always use apple seeds in the juice as they contain nitrilosides, which protect us from disease.

6oz/170g grapes
1 apple
Crushed ice (optional)

1. Process all the ingredients through the juicer.
2. Sit back and enjoy the delicious tastes!

Vibrant Apple, Carrot and Ginger

serves 1

Initially when I started juicing this was my favourite juice. The colour and taste of this juice is so vibrant that you can almost feel it doing good for you before you even drink it! Don't forget always to use the apple seeds in the juice. Carrots are rich in calcium, phosphorus, potassium, folic acid and carotonids such as beta-carotene. Ginger is powerful at aiding digestion. This juice is fantastic for both the eyes and the bones.

2 carrots
1 apple
¼-inch piece of fresh ginger (optional)

1. Wash all ingredients and process them through the juicer.

Tantalizing Pineapple, Carrot and Lemon

serves 1–2

What nicer way to hydrate your body than with this sweet-tasting juice? I don't always have the time to peel pineapples and lemons, so this juice has become a favourite 'Lazy Sunday' juice as I can afford to take the time out to make it. The lemon adds a little sharpness, which is great for waking up your taste buds. Lemons are also superb cleansers for the body. Pineapple is wonderful at repairing damaged tissue and aiding digestion.

½ lemon
½ pineapple
3 carrots

1. Peel the lemon and pineapple.
2. Place in the juicer with the carrots and process all together. It's that simple!

Sunshine Orange, Carrot and Mint

serves 1

My youngest, Julie, first tasted this juice while we were on holiday, and it has become one of her favourites since then. Oranges are rich in antioxidants, the best-known of these being vitamin C. This antioxidant, along with its many qualities of fighting infection, also protects us from free radical damage. It is particularly useful for improving iron absorption from other foods, which can be a big help to anyone who suffers from fatigue due to iron deficiency. Carrots also contain rich amounts of calcium. Mint is beneficial for colds and flu because of its antibacterial properties.

2 oranges
3 carrots
6 mint leaves (optional)

1. Peel the oranges and process with the carrots and mint leaves through the juicer. Voila!

Cool Cucumber, Celery and Lime

serves 1–2

Green juices are excellent for cleaning up digestive problems, constipation and bad breath. Because cucumbers have a high water content, they are outstanding at hydrating the body and are also superb at removing harmful substances from the bloodstream, such as uric acid. Celery is high in potassium, a good source of vitamin C and loaded with enzymes. The lime will cut through your thirst, so this is a great juice to cool you down and hydrate the body after exercise.

1 cucumber
3 stalks celery
1 lime, peeled

1. Process the cucumber and celery through the juicer.
2. Squeeze the juice of the lime into mixture.

Soothing Fennel, Carrot and Celery with Bee Pollen

serves 1–2

This is not the prettiest-looking juice, but it is packed full of goodness and definitely tastes good. Fennel is a wonderful aid for stomach cramps, water retention and for those suffering from Irritable Bowel Syndrome. It relieves wind and bloating, and is especially good at soothing the digestive system. The carrot will also help fight bacteria and viruses. Bee pollen is added because it is laden with nutrients such as carotinoids, flavonoids and phytosterols. It also adds in a touch of sweetness!

1 carrot
2 stalks celery
1 fennel bulb
1 tsp bee pollen (optional)

1. Wash all the ingredients and process through the juicer.

Lively Wheatgrass

serves 1

Learning to appreciate this juice may take some time. Drinking a small shot each day is certainly worthwhile when you consider its vast array of therapeutic benefits. Wheatgrass is very effective at detoxifying and cleansing the blood. Unfortunately, centrifugal juicers cannot juice wheatgrass so it is necessary to use a masticating juicer for this juice but it will be well worth the investment.

1 shot (2 fl oz/60ml) wheatgrass
1 stalk celery
¼-inch piece ginger
Crushed ice (optional)

1. Add all ingredients to the juicer and process!

Smoothies

*Whipped together in seconds, smoothies
are the ultimate fast food …*

The Berry Vest

serves 1

This is a good cleansing drink as blueberries are a mild laxative and are marvellous for cleaning the blood. They are also rich in antioxidants, which are very effective at improving eyesight. Apples are rich in soluble fibre which can help to relieve constipation. Kiwi is a fast-working solution to protecting us from infections from colds as they are packed with vitamin C. A lovely healthful drink with a berry delicious taste!

1 kiwi
1 apple, juiced
5oz/140g blueberries

1. Blend all ingredients together until smooth.
2. Add ice and enjoy!

It's Heaven!

serves 1

This scrumptious quick drink is excellent when you are on the run. Bananas will replenish energy levels and keep you going throughout the morning. However, they can be difficult to digest, so try to choose the fruit only when it is ripe. The mint is helpful here as it aids digestion. Try to choose red plums, as they have a higher nutrient content. Taste it – it's absolutely heavenly!

1 banana
1 plum
4 fl oz/115ml almond milk (see page 152)
Handful mint leaves (optional)

1. Blend all ingredients until smooth.
2. Add ice and enjoy!

Sneaky

serves 1

The spinach in this smoothie is a real surprise, but don't overdo it – just a small handful is enough or its strong taste will dominate. It is an easy way of sneaking uncooked green vegetables into a child's diet. Spinach is very rich in calcium and is excellent for supporting strong bones and boosting the immune system. Coconut can be useful in helping to regulate thyroid function. Trust me, this one is surprisingly good!

1 banana
4 fl oz/115ml coconut milk (tinned)
Handful spinach leaves

1. Blend all ingredients together until smooth.
2. Add ice and enjoy!

Berry Delicious

serves 1

This one is a constant favourite with my daughter Julie throughout the summer. Try always to use strawberries and raspberries when they are in season. Strawberries help promote the production of collagen, vital for healthy skin, while raspberries are useful for breaking up mucus. These berries are also a rich source of vitamin B_{17} which can help protect against cancer.

> 1 apple, juiced
> 5oz/140g strawberries
> 4oz/115g raspberries
> Handful of ice

1. Juice the apple and blend all the ingredients until the desired consistency is reached.
2. Add ice and serve!

Mmmm!

serves 1

This smoothie has an incredibly delicious taste and it is so simple to prepare. It is as close to a Piña Colada without the alcohol as you will get. Pineapple is rich in bromelain, a plant enzyme, and also has powerful immune boosting properties. It has been widely studied for its potential healing powers; it aids digestion as the bromelain helps break down protein. Coconut is rich in many nutrients such as calcium, magnesium and potassium, and is very nourishing for the nervous system. Udo's Oil is rich in essential fats that feed the brain.

> 1 pineapple, peeled
> 4 fl oz/115ml coconut milk (tinned)
> ½ tsp Udo's Oil
> Handful of ice

1. Blend all the ingredients until the desired consistency is reached.
2. Add ice and serve!

That's Lovely ...

serves 1

You just can't beat this naturally sweet drink for its impressive levels of nutrients, such as beta-carotene and vitamin C, which protect us from cell damage and reduce the risk of cancer. Oranges are a good internal antiseptic and they also help stimulate cleaning of the intestines. The lecithin helps reduce cholesterol.

1 orange, peeled and juiced
1 mango, peeled
1 tbs lecithin
1 tsp Udo's Oil

1. Blend all ingredients together until smooth.
2. Add ice and enjoy!

Strawberry Fields

serves 1

I often try out different milks such as rice milk, almond milk and coconut milk for a variety of flavours. If you have the time, why not try to make your own coconut milk? (See page 151 for recipe details.) Bananas are a rich source of phosphorus and magnesium. Try to use only ripe bananas, as unripe ones are difficult to digest and may cause constipation. Although they can be difficult to find in the shops, apricot kernels are included as they are a rich source of B_{17}. This is a superb drink to re-energize and help you get through a busy day.

> 5oz/140g strawberries
> 8 fl oz/225ml almond milk
> 1 ripe banana
> 4 apricot kernels (optional)

1. Process all ingredients through the blender.
2. Add ice and enjoy!

Breakfasts

Drizzle dairy-free milks and yoghurt over
your favourite breakfasts ...

Wild Forest Muesli

serves 1–2

Enjoy the superb energy this muesli will provide throughout the day. Sunflower seeds are particularly useful for strengthening eyesight, and the berries add such sweetness. You can vary the fruits according to season.

2oz/55g sunflower seeds, soaked and rinsed
2oz/55g pumpkin seeds, soaked and rinsed
3 dried apricots, chopped
2oz/55g raspberries
2½oz/70g blueberries

1. Soak the seeds overnight and rinse the following morning.
2. Leave to drain while you prepare the fruits.
3. Mix together and drizzle over some fresh rice milk or coconut milk.

Exotic Muesli

serves 1–2

This muesli will give you a very satisfying start to your day. It is rich in zinc, magnesium and vitamin E, a powerful antioxidant with anti-cancer properties. It is loaded with enzymes as the seeds are sprouted.

2oz/55g sunflower seeds, soaked and rinsed
2oz/55g oat groats, soaked and rinsed
4 dates, chopped
1 mango, chopped
2 kiwis, chopped
Rice milk

1. Soak the seeds and groats overnight and rinse the following morning.
2. Leave to drain while you chop the fruits.
3. Mix together and drizzle rice milk on top.

Living Granola

serves 1–2

This recipe is best prepared in a dehydrator, although it can be prepared in a fan oven at a very low temperature. The sprouted buckwheat is loaded with vitamin B_{17}. You can omit the honey if you are trying to stay away from sugars.

12oz/340g buckwheat (sprouted)
1–2 tsp cinnamon
2 tsp manuka honey

1. Mix all the ingredients together and spread onto Teflex or baking sheet.
2. Dehydrate until crunchy. If using the oven method, set your oven at the lowest temperature. Turn on the fan, half-open the oven door and dehydrate until crunchy. This of course takes much longer than the dehydrator.
3. Pour over some delicious blueberry almond yoghurt (see page 150) and serve!

Blueberry Almond Yoghurt

serves 2

This is not a true yoghurt but is absolutely mouth-watering and rich in proteins. It is a great accompaniment for muesli or granola. Use blanched almonds to save time.

> 5oz/140g almonds (blanched)
> 8 fl oz/225ml water
> 3½oz/100g blueberries
> 2 dates

1. Blend the ingredients together until smooth.
2. Serve with Exotic Muesli or Living Granola (see pages 148 and 149).

Fresh Coconut Milk

serves 2–4

I love the taste of this delicious milk. It works well poured over your favourite breakfast or combined with fruits in a smoothie. If you are lactose intolerant or you are simply trying to stay away from dairy products, this is a simple alternative.

36 fl oz/1 litre warm water
170g/6oz desiccated coconut

1. Put the coconut into the blender with half the water – just enough water to move the coconut around.
2. Once it stops moving, add more water until it becomes a smooth cream.
3. Add the rest of the water a bit at a time.
4. When the coconut is finally blended, pour into a bag (cheese cloth/muslin/nut milk bag) and sieve through.
5. The pulp will remain in the bag and can be used for biscuits, etc.
6. Serve. Alternatively, this can be stored for up to three days in the refrigerator.

Almond Milk

serves 4

Many people have very low lactase levels. The inability to absorb lactose can lead to many problems if dairy products are included in the diet. This easy-to-prepare milk is a nutritious alternative to dairy milk. Enriched with essential fats, it is truly an excellent source of nutrients.

    5oz/140g almonds, soaked overnight
    1 tsp natural vanilla essence
    54 fl oz/1½ litres water
    5 tbs Udo's Oil
    2 tbs honey

1. Blend all ingredients together and serve.

No-cook Soups

*The ultimate cup of soup – with
fresh ingredients, as nature intended ...*

Super Rich Broccoli and Almond Soup

serves 1–2

Broccoli is just perfect for this tasty uncooked soup. Its sulphur-rich compounds protect the liver and have anti-cancer and antibiotic properties. This version relies on the almonds to create a protein-rich soup. It's deliciously rich and creamy!

    5oz/140g almonds, soaked overnight
    1 head broccoli
    18 fl oz/½ litre boiling water
    ½ lemon, juiced
    2 tsp vegetable bouillon
    ¼ tsp cayenne pepper

1. Wash broccoli and chop into small chunks.
2. Add boiling water and blend.
3. Rinse and drain the almonds and add them; continue blending.
4. Add the rest of the ingredients and season to taste.

Asian Seaweed Soup

serves 2

If you enjoy seafood then you are sure to take pleasure from the fishy taste of this truly lovely uncooked soup. Seaweed is such a wonderful addition to our diet, as it is packed with minerals. This soup can be mixed together in seconds – it is the perfect instant soup. Coconut can be bought in small blocks in a healthfood shop and gives the soup a distinctive Thai flavour. *Amazing!*

4oz/115g seaweed (dulse)
1 red pepper
½ block Coconut Cream
½ avocado (optional)
10 fl oz/285ml boiling water
1 tsp tamari

1. Blend the seaweed, red pepper and coconut.
2. Add avocado, if desired, and blend.
3. Add the boiling water and tamari.
4. Serve immediately.

Fresh Tomato and Basil Soup

serves 1–2

My friend Veronica, who has amazing talents in the preparation
of delicious uncooked foods, introduced me to this tasty soup
and it has become a family favourite. The herbal appeal of the
fresh basil gives this soup its unique flavour. You can easily
increase the amounts if preparing for larger numbers. *Delicious!*

1 clove garlic
6 sun-dried tomatoes, soaked in water
1 celery stick
Handful fresh basil
Handful fresh oregano
3 tomatoes
2 tsp vegetable bouillon

1. Process the garlic, sun-dried tomatoes, celery and herbs.
2. When blended, add the tomatoes and bouillon.
3. Blend until you reach a chunky consistency.
4. Warm through at a very low heat to preserve the enzymes.
   Serve warm.

Cooked Soups

*Comforting, heart-warming soups
with added nutrition ...*

Heart-warming Protein-rich Soup

serves 2–4

There is very little preparation needed for this heart-warming antioxidant-rich soup. By adding the sprouted quinoa and seaweed at the end of preparation you can turn this soup into a really healthy, nourishing meal loaded with minerals and proteins. Trust me, it turns out perfect every time!

2 sweet potatoes

2 carrots

2 onions

2 stalks celery

2 cloves garlic

3 tsp vegetable bouillon

36 fl oz/1 litre water

2 tbs sprouted quinoa, soaked overnight and rinsed

Handful seaweed

1. Peel the sweet potatoes and wash the remaining veg. Place all the veg into a saucepan.
2. Cook for 40 minutes at a medium heat until the veg softens.
3. Add the sprouted quinoa and seaweed at the end for extra nutrients.
4. Liquidize with a hand blender and serve.

Butternut Squash, Coconut and Chilli Bean Soup

serves 2–4

A beautiful, rich, creamy soup perfected by Cornucopia's chef Sinead Curtin. The butternut squash intensifies the richness of this soup; squash is so versatile as it can be added to numerous recipes. Coconut adds a distinctive Thai taste that mingles well with the subtle but not overpowering taste of the chilli. This is a real favourite with my bunch.

1 medium butternut squash
1 medium onion
1 medium carrot
½ small red chilli
18 fl oz/500ml vegetable stock
1 tin (14 fl oz/400ml) coconut milk
Bunch basil

1. Cut butternut squash in half, leaving the skin on. Remove any seeds.
2. Bake the squash skin-side down at 400°F/200°C/GM6 until soft. Set aside to cool.
3. In a large pan, add the onion, carrot and chilli to a small amount of water and sauté gently for 10 minutes, stirring regularly to prevent the vegetables sticking.
4. Add the stock and bring to a gentle simmer, cover and cook for a further 15 minutes.
5. When cooled, peel the butternut squash and roughly chop the flesh.
6. Add the butternut squash and coconut milk to the soup and simmer for a further 10 minutes or until all the vegetables are just tender.
7. Blend the soup until smooth, adding more stock if the soup is too thick. Garnish with basil and serve.

Sweet Potato and Lemongrass Soup

serves 2–4

It is worth familiarizing yourself with this tropical grass, as it adds such wonderful Thai flavours to soups and various dishes. This recipe takes full advantage of the distinctive flavour of the lemongrass. Be sure to chop it finely and soak it in some hot water to add a real zing to the soup. The almonds not only make this super-rich in proteins but they also give it a wonderful creamy texture.

4 medium sweet potatoes, whole and in their skins

1 medium carrot, diced fine

1 medium onion, chopped fine

½ small dried red chilli

2 stalks lemongrass, chopped fine and soaked in
10 fl oz/250ml hot water

30 fl oz/750ml vegetable stock

Bunch fresh coriander

3oz/100g ground almonds

4oz/100g baby spinach for garnish

1. Prick the sweet potatoes with a fork and oven-bake at 400°F/200°C/GM6 for 30–40 minutes or until soft. Set aside to cool.
2. Add a couple of tablespoons water/stock to a large saucepan.
3. Add carrots, onion and chilli.
4. Cover and sauté gently for 10 minutes, stirring regularly to prevent the vegetables sticking.
5. Add the lemongrass, soaking liquid and the stock and bring to a gentle simmer.
6. Cover and cook for a further 15 minutes.
7. Peel the cooled sweet potatoes and roughly chop the flesh.
8. Add the sweet potato, coriander and ground almonds to the soup and blend until smooth.
9. Season to taste, ladle soup into bowls and top with a little spinach.

Fresh Main Meals

*Prepared to retain their health-giving nutrients
and delicious natural taste ...*

Vegetable Stir Raw with Ginger and Almond Dressing

serves 2

Unlike most dehydrated foods, this dish is ready to eat in a very short time. Instead of ordering a Chinese meal you can prepare your own with delicious, nutritious ingredients. Serve with Thai Parsnip Rice (see page 210).

1 clove garlic
1¼oz/35g pine nuts
1 piece ginger
1 tsp vegetable bouillon
1½ tbs lemon juice
2½ tbs olive oil
4oz/110g spinach
6oz/170g bean sprouts
3oz/85g mushrooms
1 red pepper

1. Blend the garlic, pine nuts, ginger and bouillon together.
2. Add lemon juice and oil.
3. Coat the vegetables in dressing and place in dehydrator till the vegetables become warm and slightly softened (approximately half an hour). Serve.

Unfried Italian-style Vegetables

serves 2

This popular Tuscan combination of unfried vegetables is such a tasty change from the over-cooked versions that have become the norm in modern-day cooking. The crunchy texture is wonderful. You can substitute the courgettes with peppers if you prefer. *Buon Appetito!*

5 tomatoes
½ courgette
3oz/85g green olives, pitted
4 fl oz/115ml Udo's Oil
1 tsp apple cider vinegar
1 clove garlic, crushed
Handful fresh basil leaves

1. Chop the tomatoes, courgette and pitted olives.
2. Blend the rest of the ingredients and pour over the tomato, courgette and olive mixture.
3. Place on a dehydrator tray and dehydrate at 110°F/43°C for 1 hour.
4. Alternatively, spread on a baking sheet (setting the oven at its lowest temperature), turn on the fan, half-open the oven door and dehydrate for about 2 hours.

Red Pepper Ragu Sauce

serves 2

I use this sauce for the pizza base, but it works equally well as a pasta sauce for sweet potato spaghetti. To make the spaghetti you use a spiralizer – this inexpensive handy gadget can be bought in kitchen shops. Simply peel the sweet potato and spiral – you'll have raw spaghetti in seconds. Gently warm the sauce and pour over the raw spaghetti. *Viola!*

2 cloves garlic
½ apple
1 red pepper
6 sun-dried tomatoes, soaked in water
Fresh or dried herbs (basil, oregano, parsley)
1 tsp vegetable bouillon
2 tomatoes

1. Process the garlic, apple, red pepper, sun-dried tomatoes, herbs and bouillon, adding the tomatoes last.
2. Warm the mixture and use for pizza or spaghetti.

Tasty Pizza Base

serves 2

The idea of making a pizza base really seemed not worth the effort to me, until I looked at the ingredients of the average shop-bought pizza base. When I considered the nutritional differences I decided to have a go, and it really was worth making the bit of effort after all. Packed with goodness and full of taste, with no preservatives. Although it is uncooked it really tastes like pizza, especially when topped with the Health Nut's Cream Cheese (see page 174). You can store this base at room temperature for approximately two to three weeks, or alternatively you can refrigerate for the same length of time. *Bellissimo!*

1 courgette, peeled

6oz/170g buckwheat, soaked overnight and rinsed

2 tbs olive oil

2 tsp dried basil

1 tsp dried oregano

½ tsp salt

1 tsp onion powder

¼ tsp cayenne pepper

6oz/170g flax meal (ground flaxseed/linseed)

1. In a food processor, grind the peeled courgette then add the buckwheat.
2. Add all the other ingredients except the flax meal into the oil and add to mixture.
3. Blend the flax meal into the mix. Mix well.
4. Roll on to a non-stick drying sheet.
5. Roll out to form a large round (¼-inch thickness).
6. Place in dehydrator and dehydrate for 3–4 hours at 110°F/43°C.
7. Turn over and continue to dehydrate for 2 more hours.
8. Add Red Pepper Ragu Sauce, Health Nut's Cream Cheese (see pages 171 and 174) and toppings of your choice and dehydrate for ½-1 hour.
9. Serve warm.

Health Nut's Cream Cheese

this portion will cover 2 pizza bases

I use this cream cheese to top the home-made uncooked pizza, but it also works well as a spread for sandwiches or wraps. Macadamia nuts have a lovely savoury taste but they can be quite expensive and sometimes difficult to find; you can replace them with almonds if you prefer.

> 10oz/280g macadamia nuts or almonds, soaked 15 minutes
> 5oz/140g pine nuts, soaked 15 minutes
> 1 tsp nutritional yeast flakes
> 2 tbs Udo's Oil
> 4 fl oz/115ml water
> 1 tsp miso powder (optional)
> 3 tsp lemon juice

1. Grind the nuts using a food processor and add the yeast flakes.
2. Add all the other ingredients into the oil and add this to the mixture.
3. Mix well, then divide between pizza bases.

Savoury Sweetcorn Pancakes

serves 2–3

This pancake was created by Gosia, whose nutritional expertise has been invaluable to me for this book. Fill this delectable, slightly sweet pancake with Unfried Italian-style Vegetables (see page 170) for a satisfying combination. This amount will make about three pancakes.

20–25oz/565–705g fresh or frozen sweetcorn
3oz/90g ground flax seeds
1 tomato
½ small onion
2 cloves garlic
½ orange, juiced
1 tbs vegetable bouillon

1. Process all the ingredients in a powerful blender until smooth.
2. Spread on a Teflex sheet, about ½-cm thick, and dehydrate at 110°F/43°C.
3. Turn over after about 3 hours and dehydrate until the other side is solid (another 3 hours).

East Meets West Falafel

serves 2

You can make this falafel with chickpeas or butter beans; both versions work well. I usually throw this mixture together in a few minutes if I have some garlic roasting for another dish. I leave the flavours to develop overnight and roll them together for lunch the next day. *Simple!*

> 1 (14oz/400g) tin chickpeas or butter beans
> 4 cloves garlic, roasted
> 2 tbs Udo's Oil
> 2 tsp vegetable bouillon
> 2 tbs lime juice

1. Combine all the ingredients in the food processor.
2. Roll the falafel into balls.
3. Place in dehydrator till warmed through.

Fresh Crunchy Kebabs

serves 1–2

When prepared correctly, fresh vegetables have a beautiful crunchy texture. I use lots of shallots in my dishes, they are so much milder than red or white onion. Tamari (soy sauce) is excellent for quick marinades – you simply add it to some oil. These brightly coloured kebabs are delicious served on a bed of golden couscous or with a fresh green salad.

2 tbs Udo's Oil
2 tbs tamari
2 courgettes
6 shallots
2 red peppers
1 yellow pepper
3 tomatoes
3oz/85g mushrooms

1. Prepare the marinade by mixing the oil and tamari.
2. Wash and trim the vegetables and cut into bite-sized pieces.
3. Pour the marinade over the vegetables (if possible marinade the mushrooms separately).
4. Marinate for 2 hours, drain and place on skewers.
5. Dehydrate for 2 hours, drizzle with your favourite dressing and serve.

Cooked Main Meals

A liile bit more of a challenge,
but well worth the effort ...

Pinto Bean Sweet Potato Stew with Lemon Mint Pesto

serves 4

This hearty, sustaining dish is a great one-pot dish that can help solve the dilemma of family meals. To avoid last-minute fuss, don't forget to soak the beans the night before. This stew is very welcoming on a cold winter's day. This stew takes on an exciting new characteristic with the lemon pesto.

3oz/85g pinto beans, soaked and drained
14 fl oz/400ml water
1 large onion
2 large carrots
1 stalk celery
2 cloves garlic
Pinch cinnamon
2 sweet potatoes, cubed
2 courgettes

For the lemon mint pesto
1oz/30g pine nuts
Juice of one lemon
10 mint leaves
Handful of basil
Seasoning

1. To make the pinto bean stew, cook the soaked beans in the water for 30 minutes in a large pot.
2. Add sweet potato, onion, carrots, celery, garlic and cinnamon.
3. Cook gently for 30 minutes until tender.
4. Add courgettes and simmer for 5 minutes more.
5. Meanwhile, to make the pesto, use a food processor to blend the pine nuts, lemon, mint and basil together.
6. Add a little water if necessary to make a fine paste with the seasoning.
7. Stir into the finished stew and serve immediately with brown rice or millet.

Leek Pie with Roast Garlic and Butter Bean Mash

serves 2–4

The butter bean mash adds an interesting change to this savoury, satisfying pie. I know the list is long and may tend to put the fainthearted off, but this pie makes a welcoming change on a cold winter's evening. You could also try this delicious mash as a side dish with various other recipes.

- 1 large onion, chopped fine
- 2 stalks celery, chopped fine
- ½ tsp oregano
- 1 tin (14oz/400g) chopped organic tomatoes
- 1 large leek, cut into largish chunks
- 2 large floury potatoes
- ½ tin (7oz/200g) butter beans
- 1 bulb garlic
- Splash of rice milk
- 6–8 button mushrooms
- 2oz/55g dried green lentils, soaked overnight
- 3½ fl oz/100ml water

1. Put the onion, celery, oregano, tomatoes and leek into a large casserole dish with a little water. Cook gently for 15 minutes.
2. Meanwhile, make the mash: Peel and cook the potatoes until tender and bake with the garlic at 400°F/200°C/GM6 for 20 minutes.
3. When cool enough to handle, peel and place in a bowl with the butter beans and rice milk.
4. Using a hand whisk, mix until the mash is creamy.
5. Meanwhile, bake the mushrooms at 400°F/200°C/GM6 and cook the soaked lentils in the water for 15 to 20 minutes.
6. Rinse and add the mushrooms and lentils to the veg mixture.
7. Top the mixture with the mash.
8. Smooth with a palette knife and bake for 35 minutes at 400°F/200°C/GM6 until golden brown.

Vegetable Ragout with Herb Spaghetti

serves 4

The distinctive anise flavour of the fennel shines through in this tasty vegetable ragout. This delicious dish from Margaret Burke of Cornucopia makes a refreshing change. Experiment with different pastas, such as Kamut, which is very similar in taste to the familiar durum wheat spaghetti but much easier to digest.

2 cloves garlic

1 red onion, chopped

1 fennel bulb, chopped

1 red pepper

1 yellow pepper

1 tin (14oz/400g) tomatoes, chopped

1 tsp rosemary, chopped fine

Asparagus spears (blanched) – 8 sticks sliced lengthways

4 tsp basil, chopped roughly

7oz/200g wholewheat spaghetti

1. Add garlic, onion, fennel and peppers to a large pot with a little water.
2. Fit a lid and cook gently for 15 minutes or until tender.
3. Add tomatoes and rosemary.
4. Cook gently for a further 10–15 minutes.
5. Meanwhile, blanch the asparagus in a separate pot of boiling water and set aside.
6. Remove with slotted spoon; the water can be used to cook the spaghetti.
7. Cook the spaghetti from directions on the packet.
8. Drain the spaghetti and mix into the torn basil.
9. Season the sauce, and serve the spaghetti and sauce with a few spears of asparagus on top.

Sweet Potato and Broccoli Sambar

serves 4

When you look at the list of ingredients you may think this recipe is a little complex, but the majority of ingredients are herbs and spices that most of us have in the cupboard. This sweet, rich Sambar created by Phil and Tony of Cornucopia can make an evening special. Feel free to vary it with a different range of seasonal vegetables.

Water
1 onion
2 carrots
1 red chilli
½ tsp ginger
1 tsp cumin
¼ tsp turmeric
Pinch cinnamon
1 tsp ground coriander
1 courgette
2 sweet potatoes
2oz/55g red split lentils
1 large head broccoli
Seasoning

1. In a large pot containing approximately half a pint
   (10 fl oz/285ml) of water, add the onion, carrots, chilli, ginger,
   cumin, turmeric, cinnamon and coriander.
2. Cook gently with fitted lid until vegetables are beginning to
   soften.
3. Add sweet potatoes.
4. Cook gently for 20 minutes, until vegetables are soft.
5. Meanwhile cook the lentils in 3½ fl oz/100ml of water until
   yellow (about 15–20 minutes) and set aside.
6. Blanch the broccoli.
7. Stir lentils, blanched broccoli and seasoning into cooked
   onion, carrot and spices mixture.
8. Serve poured over brown rice.

Puy Lentil and Spinach Stew

serves 2–4

Adding the spinach at the end of the cooking process gives this stew a rich amount of nutrients. The slightly wilted spinach also gives this classic stew a rich colour. I use fresh herbs generously because they add such wonderful flavours to the blandest ingredients. Serve with some baby potatoes.

3½oz/200g dried puy lentils

1 clove garlic, crushed

2 sprigs fresh thyme

2 sprigs fresh rosemary

Water

1oz/30g butter

1 medium red onion, chopped fine

2 cloves garlic, chopped fine

4 bay leaves

4oz/110g baby spinach

2 tbs cold-pressed extra virgin olive oil

1. Cook the puy lentils with the crushed garlic clove, thyme and rosemary in plenty of water.

2. Pick out the rosemary and thyme and set aside.

3. Meanwhile, melt the butter gently in a large saucepan and add the red onion, chopped garlic and bay leaves.

4. Cover and reduce heat, cooking gently for 10 minutes or until the onions are softened.

5. Turn off the heat and set aside.

6. When the puy lentils are just cooked but retain a little bite, drain the liquid, remove the garlic and add the mixture to the onions.

7. Add a couple of tablespoons of water, cover with a lid, and allow to braise for a further 10 minutes or until the lentils are tender.

8. Turn off the heat.

9. Stir in the spinach and oil, season and serve.

Tuscan-style Peppers

serves 4

It is impossible to go wrong with this impressive dish – believe me, no one will leave the table dissatisfied. They are absolutely bursting with flavour. Make sure you add the essential fats at the end of the cooking process so their essential nutrients are not destroyed by the heat. Served on a bed of crisp fresh leaves, this dish looks every bit as good as it tastes.

4 medium red peppers, halved and deseeded
1oz/30g butter
1 red onion, chopped fine
4 cloves garlic, chopped fine
2 courgettes, diced fine
2 cups organic brown rice, cooked
6oz/170g black olives, roughly chopped
2 tsp capers, roughly chopped (optional)
5oz/140g sun-dried tomatoes, soaked in hot water
    and chopped fine
Handful of torn fresh basil leaves
2 tbs Udo's Oil
Seasoning

1. Roast the peppers in a moderate oven for 20 minutes or until just tender.
2. Meanwhile, melt the butter in a pan and add the onion and garlic and cook on a low heat until softened.
3. Add the courgettes and cook for a further 5 minutes.
4. Stir in all the remaining ingredients except the oil. Season with salt and pepper and fill the peppers with this mixture.
5. Return to the oven and cook for 10–15 minutes or until heated through.
6. Remove from the oven, drizzle with oil and serve immediately with a hearty green salad.

Snacks

Mouth-watering wraps, crisps and dips ...

Fabulous Lunch Patties

serves 2

With a proper combination of papaya, avocado and garlic, these patties have a distinctive aroma after dehydrating. It might take a couple of trials to perfect this recipe, but it's definitely worth it. Celery provides a salty taste to foods, so is especially good to add to dishes if you are trying to cut back on your salt intake.

2 ripe medium papayas
1 avocado
2 cloves garlic
3 stalks celery
Pinch of ground white pepper

1. Peel the papayas and discard the seeds.
2. Put all the ingredients into the blender and process until smooth.
3. Form patties and place on a Teflex sheet. Patties should be about 1.5 cm thick, and dehydrate at 110°F/43°C.
4. Turn over after about 6 hours (when the first side is dry) and dehydrate until the other side is solid (another 3 hours).

Energy Wraps with Garlic Dill Sauce

serves 2

These wraps are very quick to prepare for a short lunch break.
Unlike sandwiches they have no extra calories from the bread.
The sauce takes about three minutes and is well worth the effort.
To save time you can prepare the sauce in advance.

1 red pepper

2 tomatoes

2 shallots

3 large lettuce leaves

6oz/170g alfalfa sprouts

5oz/140g pine nuts, soaked

1 clove garlic

2 tomatoes

½oz/15g fresh dill

½ lime, juiced

pinch sea salt

1 tsp Udo's Oil

1. Wash and chop the red pepper, tomato and shallots.
2. Fill the lettuce leaves evenly with vegetables and sprouts.
3. Blend the pine nuts, garlic, tomatoes, dill, lime juice, sea salt
   and oil in a blender or small processor all at one go! Whizz
   together and drizzle over wrap filling.
4. Roll together to form a wrap.

Corn on the Cob with Sassy Salsa

serves 2

The smoky flavour of the sun-dried tomatoes gives this spicy salsa a rich flavour and livens up the taste of the lovely, fresh corn. You could use frozen corn, but it does not have the sweetness of the fresh stuff. This is a really tasty snack, packed full of vitamins A and C.

3 fresh corn cobs
3 tomatoes
2½oz/70g sun-dried tomatoes, soaked until soft
½ chilli pepper
3 tsp apple cider vinegar
½ red pepper
Shoyu sauce
1 clove garlic

1. Strip husks from the corn by running a knife downwards to remove the kernel.
2. Wash and cut into 3 pieces, cover with boiling water, set aside and prepare the salsa.
3. Blend the remainder of ingredients until a slightly chunky consistency is reached.
4. Serve the salsa drizzled over the slightly warmed corn.

Gosia's Powerful Paté

serves 2–4

Gosia created this powerful paté. She is a wonderful advertisement for eating a raw food diet. An assortment of crackers or marinated veggies complements this chunky, flavourful paté nicely. Brazil nuts are packed with selenium, the red pepper provides an abundance of vitamin C, and both of these nutrients support the liver in detoxifying. Try the Marinated Broccoli (see page 218) with this one.

1 red pepper, chopped

1 tbs mild paprika powder

1 lemon, juiced

1 orange, juiced

5 cloves garlic

1 tsp white pepper, ground

10oz/280g Brazil nuts, soaked and rinsed

½oz/15g chives, chopped fine

1. Process all the ingredients, except the nuts and chives, in a blender.
2. Add the nuts and blend until smooth.
3. Sprinkle with chives and serve. Delicious!

Omega-rich Sprouted Sandwich

serves 2

If you are a bread lover, this sandwich will keep the hunger pangs away. It is an absolute favourite with my students and friends. It was one of the first sandwiches I began to add sprouts to as I made the transition to a healthier diet. You can use alfalfa or red clover sprouts in this one. The almond butter and omega-rich oil add a wonderful flavour to this simple but delicious sandwich.

> 4 slices wholemeal brown bread
> 1 tbs Udo's Oil
> 1 tbs almond butter
> 4 lettuce leaves, shredded
> ½ onion, chopped fine
> ½ red pepper, chopped fine
> 2 handfuls sprouts
> 1 tbs organic mayonnaise

1. Spread the sliced bread with the oil and almond butter.
2. Add the lettuce, onion, red pepper and sprouts.
3. Coat this sandwich with a generous amount of mayonnaise for extra flavour.

Zucchini Sandwiches

serves 2

If you have some leftover paté, these sandwiches are very easy to prepare. They make a filling and tasty midday snack, or alternatively can be served as an appetizing starter. You could easily bake these sandwiches if you don't have a dehydrator.

2 courgettes
8oz/225g Powerful Paté (see page 198)
3oz/85g black olives, pitted
½ red onion, chopped fine

1. Cut the courgettes into cracker-bread shaped pieces (1.5 cm thick, 10cm long).
2. Spread over the paté and decorate with olives and onion.
3. Place the sandwiches in the dehydrator and dehydrate for 1 hour at 110°F/43°C.
4. Alternatively set your oven to its lowest temperature, turn on the fan, half-open the oven door and bake for about 2 hours.

Mediterranean Flax Crackers

serves 2–3

The slightly sweet taste of these crackers with their Italian herbs give them a beautiful flavour. I use dry herbs for this cracker, but remember they are more pungent than fresh herbs so you need only small amounts. Flax seeds are included as they are an important source of fibre. Sassy Salsa (see page 197) makes a lovely accompaniment to these Italian-style crackers.

> 4oz/120g flax seeds, soaked
> 1 onion
> 1 red pepper
> 1 stalk celery
> 1 carrot
> 1 tsp basil
> 1 tsp oregano
> 4 fl oz/115ml water

1. Mix ingredients bit by bit into a masticating juicer or food processor. Process thoroughly until the mixture is well blended together. Spread the mixture fairly thin onto a Teflex drying sheet. Place in a dehydrator and dry until crisp (approximately 6 hours).

Sun-kissed Basil Pesto

serves 2

It is difficult to beat the aroma of fresh basil. Fresh basil is widely known to be a powerful aphrodisiac; the herb provides a pungent smell to this magnificent pesto. Pine nuts have a rich oily texture that helps when blending this mix together.

1 clove garlic
1 fresh yellow bell pepper
2 medium tomatoes
5oz/140g pine nuts, soaked for 1 hour
1oz/30g fresh basil
½ lime, juiced
1 tsp Udo's Oil

1. Peel the garlic clove and wash the vegetables.
2. Blend all the ingredients in a blender until smooth.
3. Can be served with pasta.

Ripe Guacamole Dip

serves 2–4

I like to include avocados in my diet because they protect the body from free radical damage and are a good source of vitamins C and E. It should be noted that avocados discolour quickly, so it is best to add the lemon juice into the mixture as soon as you peel the avocado. Why not try them with some Spicy Curry Crackers (see page 204)?

2 ripe avocados
1 clove garlic
1 shallot
1 lemon, juiced
1 tsp Udo's Oil
Handful of red clover sprouts (optional)

1. Peel the avocados and remove the stones.
2. Place in a small processor with the other ingredients. Blend until smooth and serve immediately.

Spicy Curry Crackers

serves 2–4

These crackers are delicious served with a nut cheese or guacamole dip. Don't be put off by the amount of ingredients involved. Once you remember to soak the seeds and almonds, the rest is straightforward.

2½oz/70g almonds, soaked

3 carrots

1 onion

5 stalks celery

2oz/60g parsley

1 lemon, juiced

4 tbs curry powder

12oz/340g flax seeds, soaked

1. Process all the ingredients, except the flax seeds, through a food processor.
2. Add the flaxseeds and mix well.
3. Spread on a Teflex sheet, ½-cm thick, and form crackers with a spatula.
4. Dehydrate at 110°F/43°C for 3 hours, then turn over.
5. Remove crackers from the Teflex sheet and place direct on dehydrator tray; continue dehydrating for another 8 hours at the same temperature.

Get Stuffed Tomatoes

serves 2

Stuffed tomatoes are very satisfying for a light lunch, or if combined with a large salad will satisfy the heartiest of appetites. The wonderful combination of flavours of the sun-kissed pesto is absolutely heavenly. They can be dehydrated for 1 hour if you prefer something warm, or eaten in their raw state. Either way works well.

> **3 large tomatoes**
> **½ red onion**
> **8oz/225g Sun-kissed Pesto (see page 202)**
> **½oz/15g fresh parsley**

1. Cut the tomatoes into halves and scoop out pulp from the centres.
2. Chop the onion.
3. Fill the tomato halves with pesto and sprinkle with red onion and parsley.

Hearty Stuffed Mushrooms

serves 2

These are my absolute favourite – hands down. The stuffing for these mushrooms is truly delicious and very substantial. I find that the minute they are prepared they disappear quickly – especially when my son Richard is around! If you need some inspiration, this satisfying dish is uncomplicated and delicious.

12 mushrooms, cleaned

2 fl oz/60ml shoyu sauce

2 fl oz/60ml olive oil

2½oz/70g pine nuts

4 cherry tomatoes

1 tsp onion powder

1 tbs Udo's Oil

Fresh herbs (basil, oregano, sage)

1. Clean the mushrooms and marinate in the shoyu sauce and olive oil for 20 minutes, tossing gently occasionally.
2. Process the nuts, tomatoes and onion powder, adding the Udo's Oil last.
3. Stuff each mushroom with approximately half a teaspoon of the mixture.
4. Place in dehydrator for 1–2 hours.

Sides

Quick and easy …

No-grain Tabbouleh

serves 2

This tabbouleh is completely grain free, and excellent for people on a gluten-free diet. Unlike tabbouleh made from bulgar, which can be difficult to digest, this version is very easily digested and is a nice accompaniment to any dish. Fresh parsley and lemon juice ensure a wonderful depth of flavour to this simple but tasty dish. A nice one to add to your repertoire.

½ cauliflower
½ red pepper
4oz/120g parsley chopped
1 lemon, juiced
2 tsp vegetable bouillon

1. Chop the cauliflower finely in a food processor.
2. Chop the red pepper into small pieces.
3. Chop the parsley finely.
4. Combine together with the lemon juice and bouillon.

Thai Parsnip Rice

serves 2–3

This simple rice is invaluable if you are tired of cooking. I first ate a similar version of this rice at an exquisite meal prepared by the talented chef Chad Sarrno. This simple version has been a big hit with my friends and students, not only for its taste but because it is so easy to prepare. It is also delicious when served with a fresh green salad.

> 2 parsnips
> 1¼oz/35g pine nuts, soaked
> 2 tsp Udo's Oil

1. Peel the parsnips and chop with the nuts in a processor.
2. Add oil and place on parchment paper in dehydrator until warm (approximately half an hour).
3. Serve with warmed Vegetable Stir Raw (see page 169).

Golden Couscous

serves 1–2

Couscous is one of the easiest grains to prepare. I use turmeric and lemon juice in this version to give it its nice golden colour. Turmeric is rich in curcumin, which has been found to have potent anti-cancer properties. Parsley adds a nice splash of colour to the dish, and is useful for reducing gallstones and kidney stones. By growing a few herbs on the kitchen windowsill you will have a constant supply at hand to snip and add to dishes.

½ tsp turmeric
½ lemon, juiced
6oz/170g couscous
Water, boiling, to cover
2oz/60g parsley

1. Combine turmeric and lemon juice together in a small saucepan.
2. Pour in couscous and cover with enough boiling water to barely cover the couscous. Leave for 10 minutes until the water is absorbed.
3. Stir in the chopped parsley and serve warm or cold.

Salads

Scrumptious and inviting ...

Mixed Herb Salad
with Spicy Sunflower Seeds

serves 2

The wonderful flavours of the fresh herbs in this salad make it an absolute winner. The spicy seeds can be added to the salad or eaten on their own. Parsley is packed with iron and magnesium and is marvellous for anybody suffering from anaemic conditions. Basil is my favourite of all herbs, and I use it in abundance, while sunflower seeds protect us from infection.

> 3 tbs sunflower seeds
> 1 tbs Udo's Oil
> ½ tsp curry powder
> 12oz/340g mixed salad leaves
> 12oz/340g mixed herbs (basil and parsley)
> 2 shallots, chopped fine

1. Soak the seeds in the oil and curry powder, allowing them to pick up the flavour of the curry.
2. Mix together the salad leaves, herbs and shallots.
3. Drizzle over your favourite dressing and sprinkle with the spicy sunflower seeds.

Crisp Baby Spinach Leaves with Garlic Mushrooms

serves 1–2

You may not like the smell of garlic, but even if you're not inclined to use garlic give these mushrooms a try. I use the dehydrator for these mushrooms as it intensifies their flavour. Buy the freshest looking organic leaves you can get your hands on to ensure that the salad is nice and crispy. Spinach is packed with nutrients and is especially good served with these scrumptious mushrooms.

> 12oz/340g mushrooms
> 8 fl oz/225ml cup Udo's Oil
> 4 cloves garlic, crushed
> 12oz/340g spinach leaves
> 12oz/340g mixed leaves

1. Wash, slice and coat the mushrooms with the oil and crushed garlic.
2. Place in dehydrator for 1 hour. If you do not have a dehydrator, slice the mushrooms thinly and marinate overnight.
3. Wash and prepare the leaves.
4. Drizzle over some oil and add mushrooms.

Slurpy Tomato and Onion Salad

serves 1–2

Choose some nice juicy ripe tomatoes for this easy-to-prepare salad. Onions are amazing at removing parasites from the body and are also a good source of folic acid. The turmeric doesn't overpower this juicy dish, which is delicious served with Golden Couscous (see page 211). It is both attractive and delicious!

> 5 tomatoes
> 1 red onion, chopped fine
> 4 tsp tamari
> 6 dessertspoons apple cider vinegar
> 4 dessertspoons cold-pressed olive oil
> 1 tsp turmeric
> Basil, chopped

1. Wash and slice tomatoes. Arrange them, with the onion, on a dish.
2. Mix the tamari, vinegar, oil and turmeric together and pour over the onion and tomato. Allow to marinate for 5–10 minutes.
3. Sprinkle with chopped basil before serving.

Marinated Broccoli with Sprouted Sesame Seeds

serves 4

Served as a side salad, or used with dips, this dish provides high amounts of powerful protective nutrients including selenium, magnesium, vitamin C and folic acid. All of the aforementioned are anti-cancer and liver-friendly nutrients that boost the liver's ability to detoxify. Marinating the broccoli will ensure a much better depth of flavour.

1 head broccoli
4 fl oz/115ml Udo's Oil and olive oil (50:50)
1 lemon, juiced
Sea salt for taste optional
3 tsp sesame seeds (sprouted)

1. Chop the broccoli into small florets.
2. Mix the oils, lemon juice and sea salt to taste; toss the broccoli in this marinade until well coated.
3. Cover and marinate overnight in the refrigerator.
4. Toss the sprouted sesame seeds over the marinated broccoli.
5. Serve with Gosia's Powerful Paté (see page 198).

No-cook Tasty Treats

Nutritious and guilt-free …

Lovely Love Bites

serves ? – it's up to you!

'Love at first bite' is the best way to describe the delectable alluring taste of these tempting treats. They are so *mmmm* you may not want to share them. They are perfect after a meal. Rather than using the zest of the orange, I peel the skin, leaving the white pith behind. This gives these love bites a real tasty zing. They are positively *seductive!*

> 1 orange, peeled and juiced
> 10oz/280g almonds, soaked and rinsed
> 5oz/140g raisins, soaked in orange juice
> 1½oz/45g millet, soaked and rinsed
> 3oz/85g desiccated coconut

1. Chop the peeled orange skin in a processor.
2. Blend all ingredients except the coconut through the juicer or processor. Roll out into balls and coat each ball in coconut.
3. Refrigerate for 1 hour.

Instant Sticky Fudge

serves 2–4

This fudge will get you out of a sticky situation if your sweet tooth demands some attention – so be sure to keep some on hand. It is the perfect antidote for the sugar blues. But be warned … one just won't be enough.

18oz/510g desiccated coconut
2oz/55g carob powder
3 tbs honey
2 tsp lecithin granules
1 tsp natural vanilla essence

1. Process all ingredients together.
2. Press into a shallow dish and chill.
3. Cut into squares before serving.

Heavenly Divine Nectar

serves 2–4

When served with Zesty Walnut Munchies (see page 227), this heavenly mousse makes a delicious mouth-watering treat. This is a nice way of using up leftover ripe bananas – it's a good idea always to peel and freeze leftover bananas, as they can be extremely handy for making ice creams, smoothies and other desserts. *Divine!*

> 3 bananas, peeled and frozen
> 1 ripe mango
> 2 dates

1. Process all ingredients in food processor.
2. Serve immediately.

Pam's Pudding

serves 2–3

You are sure to enjoy the texture of this pudding. It is the avocado that gives it its rich, creamy texture. You can also add some chopped nuts to this pudding, though I prefer the delicate taste of mint. Mint should only be added just before serving, as the leaves tend to blacken once cut. This can easily be prepared in advance.

> 2 bananas, peeled and frozen
> 10oz/280g strawberries
> ½ avocado
> 4 fl oz/115ml water
> Mint leaves, chopped

1. Combine all the ingredients in food processor.
2. Spoon into small serving dishes and chill for 1 hour.
3. Decorate with chopped mint and serve.

Healthy Ice Cream with Caramelized Pecans

serves 2

With *no* colourings or artificial flavourings, this scrumptious potassium-rich ice cream is a wonderful nutritious treat. I promise you it won't last very long! The caramelized pecans are incredibly easy to prepare. *Yummy!*

3 bananas, peeled and frozen
5oz/140g frozen strawberries
2 dates, pitted
2oz/55g pecans, chopped
1 tbs agave syrup
1 tsp tamari

1. Mix the bananas, strawberries and dates together in a food processor.
2. Coat the chopped pecans in agave syrup and tamari.
3. Sprinkle over the ice cream and serve immediately.

Mango and Coconut Ice Cream

serves 2–4

It is evident from the deep orange colour of mangoes that they are a rich source of beta-carotene. The flavours of mango and coconut contrast beautifully in this delicious ice cream. A good food processor will reduce the preparation time of this ice cream to a minimum. Enjoy!

2 ripe mangoes
Zest and juice of 1 lime
Sea salt
1 tsp honey
2 fl oz/60ml coconut milk

1. Peel and chop the mangoes into 3-cm pieces and freeze on a flat tray lined with baking parchment for 2 hours.
2. Put the frozen mango into a food processor and blend on pulse to a puree.
3. Add the lime zest and juice, a pinch of salt and the honey (if required).
4. While the food processor is running, add the coconut milk.
5. Pour the mix into a suitable container and freeze for half an hour.
6. Serve.

Zesty Walnut Munchies

serves 4

One bite of these delicious munchies and you will be hooked. When I make a plate of these for my daughter Julie's friends … they disappear in seconds. It's the lemon peel that gives them a real zing. Try not to be put off by the length of the dehydration time. I just love their simplicity. *Zesty!*

1 lemon
12oz/340g walnuts
5oz/140g dates

1. Peel the lemon and retain the peel.
2. Juice the lemon and pour over walnuts and dates. Allow to soak overnight.
3. Grind the lemon peel finely in a food processor.
4. Add the juicy walnuts and dates to the lemon peel.
5. Process all ingredients together.
6. Press the mixture onto a board, cut into cookie shapes, place in the dehydrator overnight.

Raw Soul Apple Pie

serves 6–8

This mouth-watering creation by the brilliant chefs Lillian and Eddie Robinson will get your taste buds going. Their Raw Soul restaurant in New York is worth a visit to sample their cuisine if you're passing that way. This is the easiest apple pie I have ever prepared – no dehydrating, no cooking, just a food processor, assemble it together and *Viola!*

9oz/255g walnuts

15oz/425g almonds

15 dates, pitted

¼ tsp nutmeg

6 medium apples

10oz/280g raisins

3 tbs psyllium

½ lemon, juiced

10oz/280g almonds

8 fl oz/225ml water

1 fl oz/30ml agave syrup or 12 pitted dates, soaked

1 tsp ground cloves

1. To make the pie crust, process the walnuts, almonds, dates and nutmeg to form a fine crumb mixture.
2. Set aside 1 cup of the mixture for the top of the pie.
3. Press remaining mixture into a 9-inch glass pie dish.
4. To make the pie filling, shred the apples in a food processor and place in a large bowl.
5. Add raisins, psyllium and lemon juice and mix well.
6. Blend remaining ingredients together till smooth and creamy.
7. Add to the apple mixture, mix and pour into the pie crust. Top with the remaining cup of crumb mixture.
8. Slice and serve.

Kevin's Lemon Cheesecake

serves 6–8

My dear friend Kevin Jacobson perfected this amazing nutritious cheesecake. Kevin touched my life with his vision for embracing change. I have included this recipe for those of you who are a bit more adventurous. It is an ideal treat for a special occasion. You can also add your favourite flavouring to this recipe. A real treat without sin.

2oz/55g Carrageen (Irish moss)

5 fl oz/140ml water

11oz/310g desiccated coconut

30 fl oz/850ml water

2 fl oz/60ml honey

6 dessertspoons lecithin granules

Juice of 1 lemon

Zest of 1 lemon

1. Steep the Carrageen overnight then rinse three times, rubbing it during the rinsing.
2. Pour into a high-speed blender with the water and blend thoroughly.
3. Strain liquid through muslin/cheesecloth. Discard the pulp.
4. Soak the coconut with the warm water for a few minutes and then blend.
5. Once blended, strain through muslin/cheesecloth. Leave pulp aside.
6. In the blender, add the rest of the ingredients, plus the liquid from the seaweed and the coconut milk. Blend thoroughly.
7. Pour into a mould.
8. Store in the refrigerator for a minimum of 4 hours.
9. Serve and enjoy.

Delicious Nutritious Cookies

serves 2–3

These nutritious cookies will disappear the minute you put them on the plate! The majority of biscuits available in supermarkets contain hydrogenated or partially hydrogenated oils – these harmful fats are most definitely best avoided and these uncooked cookies are a delicious and nutritious alternative. A real favourite with my two girls. *Scrummy!*

5oz/140g almonds
6oz/170g figs
1 orange, juiced and peeled

1. Mix ingredients a bit at a time, alternating ingredients, into a masticating juicer or food processor.
2. Spread the mixture onto a chopping board and cut into shapes with a cookie cutter.
3. Place in dehydrator for 6–8 hours or until dry.
4. Turn occasionally to allow the cookies to dry evenly on both sides.

Baked Treats

*Add 'just' a little sweetness
into your life …*

Coconut Apricot Cookies

serves 2–4

I use coconut in a lot of my recipes. I love its taste and it works well with soups, main dishes and various combinations of cookies, tarts and ice creams. It is so easy to work with you just can't go wrong!

1lb/455g desiccated coconut
4oz/115g potato flour
4oz/115g soya flour
10oz/285g honey
3½ fl oz/100ml coconut oil
10oz/285g dried apricots
3½ fl oz/100ml apple concentrate

1. Mix the dry ingredients together in a bowl.
2. In a separate bowl mix the honey, coconut oil, apricots and apple concentrate.
3. Pour into the flour mixture and work into a soft dough.
4. Divide the dough into 16 portions, roll each into a ball and flatten into cookie shapes approximately 1 cm thick.
5. Bake on a greased and lined baking tray in a preheated oven 350°F/180°C/GM4 for 10–15 minutes until lightly golden brown.
6. Makes 16 cookies.

Taftans

serves 2–4

These taftans are the creation of Cornucopia's talented chef Clare McCormick. Their preparation time is minimal and their splendid savoury taste combines well with pasta and mops up the sauce nicely. You can vary the herbs according to the season.

27 fl oz/760ml water
1½ tsp dried baker's yeast
1lb/455g brown rice flour
2oz/55g coriander, chopped fine
4oz/115g red onion, chopped fine
1½oz/45g melted butter

1. First warm the water just to lukewarm (no more than 95°F/35°C).
2. Add the yeast to the water and leave until the yeast froths over the surface of the liquid.
3. In a separate bowl mix all the dry ingredients together, then pour in the yeast liquid and melted butter.
4. Mix to a thick paste-like consistency.
5. Spoon the mix onto a baking tray lined with parchment paper.
6. Make little patties approximately 1 cm thick and 8 cm wide.
7. Bake in a preheated oven 350°F/180°C/GM4 for 15 minutes or until lightly golden.
8. Makes approximately 16 biscuits.

Pumpkin Seed Bread

serves 2–4

The list of nutritious seeds in this bread make it a real winner. It's particularly hard to beat this fresh homemade bread with its pleasant crunchy taste. Simple to make but full of nutrients, flax seeds are high in fibre, pumpkin seeds are rich in calcium, B vitamins and essential fatty acids.

12oz/340g brown spelt flour

1 tbs sesame seeds

1 tbs poppy seeds

1 tbs linseeds

2 tbs sunflower seeds

2 tbs pumpkin seeds

3 tsp gluten-free baking powder

21 fl oz/600ml organic soya milk

Juice of half a lemon

1 dessertspoon treacle

1. Mix all the dry ingredients together, sieving the baking powder into the dry mix.
2. Mix the soya milk and lemon juice, add with the treacle to the dry mixture and mix thoroughly until a thick consistency is reached (similar to thick porridge).
3. Lightly coat a 450-g loaf tin with a small amount of butter and pour the mixture in. The tin should be about three-quarters full.
4. Bake in a preheated oven, 350°F/180°C/GM4 for between 45 minutes and 1 hour.
5. When tipped out, the base of the loaf should be reasonably firm.

White Spelt Yeast Bread with Millet

serves 2–4

White bread is a big favourite for many people. This version was given to me by the talented master baker George Heist. Millet is considered to be one of the most digestible and least allergenic grains. It's comprised of approximately 15 per cent protein and is rich in magnesium, phosphorus, potassium and phytochemicals.

18oz/510g white spelt flour
3½oz/100g flaked millet
¾oz/20g millet seeds
¾oz/20g fresh yeast
½oz/15g salt
11–14 fl oz/300–400 ml water

1. Mix the flour, millet and seeds in a bowl, make a dent in the centre and crumble the yeast into it.
2. Take some of the water, warm it slightly and cover the yeast.
3. Leave to ferment for approximately 20 minutes.
4. Take the fermented mixture and add the rest of the water – little by little, as you may not need all of it.
5. Mix the bread by hand, kneading the mixture until it stops sticking to the bowl or your work surface, but for at least 5–7 minutes.
6. Use a little extra flour for dusting the bowl, surface and baking tray.
7. Divide the dough into two and leave it to sit (prove) on your baking tray covered with a tea towel until it nearly doubles in size.
8. To get a nice crust it is important to wet the surface of the bread by spraying some water on top (or gently brushing it with water).
9. Place the two loaves in a preheated oven at 350°F/180°C/GM4 for approximately 40 minutes.
10. The bread should sound hollow if tapped on the bottom.

Fig and Banana Tart

serves 4–6

This beautiful tart is wonderful served warm with some Healthy Ice Cream (see page 225). Figs are an amazing natural sweetener which help to increase vitality. They are one of the richest plant sources of calcium and are also rich in phosphorus, potassium, beta-carotene and vitamin C.

1lb/455g dried figs

Water as needed

1lb/455g ripe bananas sliced approximately ½-cm thick

8oz/225g organic wholemeal flour

4oz/115g butter

Salt as needed

1 fl oz/30ml water

1. To make the filling, place the figs into a pot and pour over enough water just to cover them.
2. Bring the water to the boil and simmer the figs until they are plump.
3. While still warm, add the sliced banana, mix well and set aside.
4. To make the pastry, rub the flour, butter and salt together to make a crumbly consistency.
5. Add the water little by little and gently mix by hand until just combined.
6. Let this mixture rest in the fridge for 20 minutes.
7. Roll onto a 28-cm tart tin and rest in the fridge for a further 10 minutes.
8. Blind bake the pastry and, when ready, pour the fig/banana mix into the pastry base and smooth over.
9. Bake in a preheated oven 350°F/180°C/GM4 for 15 minutes.
10. Slice and serve.

Real Bickies

serves 2–4

The wonderful aroma of these real bickies wafting through the house brings me right back to my mother's kitchen. If you want to have a treat, these are hard to resist.

> 1lb/455g toasted whole almonds
> 12oz/340g spelt flour
> 1½ tbs gluten-free baking powder
> 1 level teaspoon salt
> 1 tsp ground cinnamon
> 10oz/285g honey
> Zest of 4 oranges
> Zest of 3 lemons
> 5 fl oz/140ml orange flower water

1. Mix the dry ingredients in a bowl and add the honey, zests and flower water.
2. Mix gently to a reasonably firm dough.
3. Cut into rounds approximately ½ cm thick and 10 cm wide.
4. Bake on a greased and lined baking tray in a preheated oven 350°F/180°C/GM4 for 10–15 minutes or until turning light golden brown.
5. Makes approximately 20 biscuits.

Resources

Naturalife Health Ltd
Rathnew
Ireland
Tel: 0404 62444
nl@naturalife.ie
www.naturalife.ie

Main stockists of Green Star masticating juicers, water distillers, dehydrators, Udo's Choice Oil Blend, Udo's Digestive Enzymes Super 8 & 5, plus speciality supplements and organic seeds for sprouting

Savant Distribution Ltd
Quarry House
Clayton Wood Close
Leeds LS16 6QE
UK
Tel: 08450 60 60 70
info@savant-health.com
www.savant-health.com

Masticating juicers, water distillers and reverse-osmosis systems, Udo's Choice Oil Blend, Udo's Digestive Enzymes Super 8 & 5, plus speciality supplements and organic seeds for sprouting

Raw Pleasure
174 Peninsula Drive
Bilimbal Heights
NSW 2486
Australia
Tel: 800-729838
www.raw-pleasure.com

Masticating juicers

Connoisseurs Australia Pty Ltd.
6 Stringer Place
Oatlands
NSW 2117
Australia
Tel: 61-2-9898-0681
www.connoisseurs.com.au

Masticating juicers

Vita-mix Corporation
8615 Usher Road
Cleveland
Ohio 44138
USA
Tel: 001 440 235 4840
Fax: 001 440 235 3726
www.vitamix.com

Powerful blenders (with European distribution)

Reverse Osmosis Ltd
Brid-A-Crinn
Dundalk
Co. Louth
Ireland
Tel: 0872 473 173
business@reverseosmosis.ie
www.reverseosmosis.ie

Eddie Daly
Grandie Marketing
255 Main Road
Dunston
Northampton NN5 6PR
Tel: 01604 752838
Fax: 01604 583997
grandie01@talk21.com

Flora Inc.
PO Box 73
805 East Badger Road
Lynden, WA 98264
US
Tel: 1-800-446 2110
www.floralhealth.com

Reverse-osmosis systems and dehydrators, distributors of Udo's products

Safe Personal-Care Products

Forever Natural UK
The Old Barrel Store
Brewery Courtyard
Drayman's Lane
Marlow, Bucks SL7 2FF
UK
Tel: 01628 891700
Fax: 01628 891701

Elysia Natural Skin Care
27 Stockwood Business Park
Stockwood
Redditch, Worcs B96 6SX
UK
Tel: 01386 792622
Fax: 01386 792623
enquiries@drhauschka.co.uk
www.drhauschka.co.uk

Neways International Ltd
12 Harvard Way
Harvard Industrial Estate
Kimbolton
Huntingdon, Cambridgeshire PE28 ONN
UK
Tel: 01480 861764
Fax: 01480 861769
info@neways.co.uk
www.neways.co.uk

The Natural Medicine Company
Burgage
Blessington
Co Wicklow
Ireland
Tel: 045 865575
Fax: 045 865827
skelly@naturalmedicine.ie

Dr Hauschka Skin Care
Heaven and Earth Ltd
3A Abbey Road
Monkstown
Co Dublin
Tel: 01284 3333
Fax: 01284 3153
info@drhauschka.ie
www.drhauschka.ie

Stockists of My Chelle Skin Care

La Sante Health Store
Dun Laoghaire Shopping Centre
Co Dublin
Tel: 01-2302090

Natural Selection

7 Seafield Road

Blackrock

Co Dublin

Tel: 01-2196980

paula@naturalselection.ie

www.naturalselection.ie

La Sante Health Store

6 Esmond Street

Gorey

Co Wexford

Tel. 055-21007

Organic Food Delivery Services

The Fresh Food Company

Tel: 020 8749 8778

www.freshfood.co.uk

Denis Healy Organic Delights

Talbotstown

Kiltegan

Co. Wicklow

Ireland

Tel: 059-6473193

info@organicdelights.ie

Absolutely Organic

Tel: 01 4600467

info@absolutelyorganic.ie

www.absolutelyorganic.ie

Wheatgrass Supplier

Living Green

Ballinclea

Donard

Co Wicklow

Tel/Fax: 045404 683

mornalynn@gmail.com

Healing Centre

Hippocrates Health Institute
1443 Palmdale Court
West Palm Beach, FL 33411
US
Tel: 561 471 8876
www.hippocrates.inst.com

Useful Websites

www.voice.buz.org
www.irishlivingfoods.com
www.cancerdecisions.com
www.changesimply.com

Bibliography and Recommended Reading

Carol Alt, *Eating in the Raw* (Clarkson Potter, 2004)

Dr Stephen and Gina Antczak, *Cosmetics Unmasked* (Thorsons, 2001)

Brendan Brazier, *Thrive* (Oceanside, 2004)

Lucy Burney, *Immunity Foods for Healthy Kids* (Duncan Baird, 2004)

Gabrielle Chavez, *The Raw Gourmet* (Findhorn, 2005)

Brian Clements, *Living Foods for Optimum Health* (Prima Health, 1998)

Alissa Cohen, *Living on Live Food* (Cohen, 2004)

Dr Rosy Daniel, *The Cancer Directory* (Thorsons, 2005)

————, *Eat to Beat Cancer* (Thorsons, 2003)

Phillip Day, *Food for Thought* (Credence Publications, 2001)

————, *Cancer: Why we're still dying to know the truth* (Credence, 1999)

Vicki Edgson and Ian Marber, *The Food Doctor* (Collins & Brown, 1999)

Udo Erasmus, *Fats that Heal, Fats that Kill* (Alive Books, 1993)

Barry Groves, *Fluoride Drinking Ourselves to Death* (Gill & Macmillan, 2001)

Siegfried Gursche, *Juicing – for the Health of It* (Alive Books, 2000)

————, *Encyclopaedia of Natural Healing* (Alive Books, 1997)

David Leggett, *Recipes for Self-Healing* (Meridian Press, 1999)

Lono Kahuna Kupua A'O, *Don't Drink the Water* (Kali Press, 1996)

Beth McEoin, *Boost Your Immune System Naturally* (Carlton, 2001)

Lynne Melcombe, *Health Hazards of White Sugar* (Alive Books, 2000)

Dr Mercola, *Total Health* (Mercola.*com*, 2004)

Kathleen O'Bannon, *Sprouts* (Alive Books, 2000)

Jane Plant, *Your Life in Your Hands* (Virgin, 2000)

Tonita d'Raye, *What's the Big Deal About Water?* (The Ten Minute Read Company, Oregon, 1995)

Rhio, *Hooked on Raw* (Beso Entertainment, 2000)

Robin Robertson, *Vegan Planet* (Harvard Common Press, 2003)

David Steinman and Samuel S. Epstein, *The Shoppers' Bible* (Wiley Publishing Inc., 1995)

P. M. Taubert, *Silent Killers – more than you paid for* (CompSafe Consultancy, 2001)

Pat Thomas, *Cleaning Yourself to Death* (Gill & Macmillan, 2001)

Jason Vale, *Slim 4 Life* (Thorsons, 2002)

————, *The Juice Master's Ultimate Fast Food* (ThorsonsElement, 2003)

Dr Norman Walker, *Water Can Undermine Your Health* (Norwalk Press, 1995)

Andrew Weil, *Spontaneous Healing* (Little Brown, 1995)

Caroline Wheater, *Juicing for Health* (Thorsons, 2001)

To contact Bernadette Bohan: b@changesimply.com

Index of Recipes

Also by Bernadette Bohan:

The Choice

*The True Story of a Mother Fighting for Her Life –
and Her Child*

In 1988 Bernadette won a battle against cancer. But when she became pregnant seven years later, a doctor told her that it was likely to trigger a return of the disease. She didn't hesitate.

Bernadette gave birth to the child she longed for. However, her fight wasn't over. Five years later, the cancer attacked her body again.

Bernadette made another choice. In desperation, she decided her best chance of survival was not simply to be the passive patient and blindly follow her doctor's advice, but to create her own alternative prescription.

When news of Bernadette's triumph over cancer brought others flocking to her door seeking help, this ordinary Irish wife and mother found her life transformed. And she realized that her sickness was a gift after all.